Medical Mnemonics

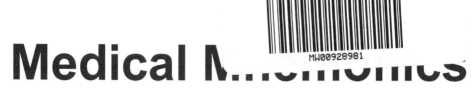

Train the brain

Mohd. Farook
M.Pharma (Pharm. Chemistry),PGDCA

Miraculous for Medical ,Para-Medical,Pharmacy and other Medical
Pre-Medical Releted competitive exams

Contents

Skin Layer
Can little girl Speak german
- S. Corneum
- S. Lucidum
- S. Granulosum
- S. Spinosum
- S. Germinative

Atrioventricular valves
"**LAB RAT**":
Left **A**trium: **B**icuspid
Right **A**trium: **T**ricuspid

Bowel components
Dow **J**ones **I**ndustrial **A**verage **C**losing **S**tock **R**eport":
From proximal to distal:
Duodenum
Jejunum
Ileum
Appendix
Colon
Sigmoid
Rectum

Diaphragm apertures: spinal levels
Aortic hiatus = **12** letters = **T12**
Oesophagus = **10** letters = **T10**
Vena cava = **8** letters = **T8**

Duodenum: lengths of parts

"Counting **1 to 4** but staggered":

1st part: **2** inches
2nd part: **3** inches
3rd part: **4** inches
4th part: **1** inch

Meckel's diverticulum details

2 inches long.
2 feet from end of ileum.
2 times more common in men.
2% occurrence in population.
2 types of tissues may be present.
Note: "**di-**" means "**two**", so **di**verticulum is the thing with all the **two**s.

Aortic arch: major branch order

"Know your **ABC'S**":
Aortic arch gives rise to:
Brachiocephalic trunk
left**C**ommon **C**arotid
left**S**ubclavian

Beware though trick question of 'What is first branch of aorta?'
Technically, it's the coronary arteries.

Aorta vs. vena cava: right vs. left

Aorta and **right** each have **5** letters, so aorta is on the right.
Vena and **cava** and **left** each have **4** letters, so vena cava is on the left.

Axillary artery branches

"Screw The Lawyer Save APatient":
Superior thoracic
Thoracoacromiol
Lateral thoracic
Subscapular
Anterior circumflex humeral
Posterior circumflex humeral
Alternatively: "Some Times Life Seems APain".

Brachial artery: recurrent and collateral branches

"IAm Pretty Sexy"
Inferior ulnar collateral artery goes with Anterior ulnar recurrent artery.
Posterior ulnar recurrent artery goes with Superior ulnar collateral artery.
   Alternatively: "IAm Pretty Smart".

External carotid artery branches

"Some Anatomists LikeF*#king, Others Prefer S&M":
Superior thyroid
Ascending pharyngeal
Lingual
Facial
Occipital
Posterior auricular
Superficial temporal
Maxillary
   Alternatively: As She LayFlat, Oscar's Passion Slowly Mounted".

Femoral triangle: arrangement of contents

NAVEL:
From lateral hip towards medial **navel**:
Nerve (directly behind sheath)
Artery (within sheath)
Vein (within sheath)
Empty space (between vein and lymph)
Lymphatics (with deep inguinal node)
Nerve/Artery/Vein are all called Femoral.

Heart valve sequence
"**Try Pul**ling **MyAorta**":
Tricuspid
Pulmonary
Mitral
Aorta

Inferior vena cava tributaries

"**I**Like **T**o **R**ise **S**o **H**igh":
Illiacs
Lumbar
Testicular
Renal
Suprarenal
Hepatic vein.
Think of the IVC wanting to rise high up to the heart.

Internal iliac artery: anterior branches

What Bill admitted to Hilary: "**IM**ilked **O**ur **I**nsatiable **I**ntern's **U**dders **U**nder the **D**esk":

Inferior gluteal
Middle rectal
Obturator
Inferior vesical artery
Internal pudendal artery
Umbilical
U/D=Uterine artery (female)/ Deferential artery (male)

Internal jugular vein: tributaries

"**M**edical **S**chools **L**et **C**onfident **P**eople **I**n":
  From inferior to superior:
Middle thyroid
Superior thyroid
Lingual
Common facial
Pharyngeal
Inferior petrosal sinus

Liver: side with ligamentum venosum/ caudate lobe vs. side with quadrate lobe/ ligamentum teres

"**VC** goes with **VC**":

The **V**enosum and **C**audate is on same side as **V**ena **C**ava [posterior].
Therefore, quadrate and teres must be on anterior by default.
  See diagram.

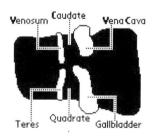

Lung lobe numbers: right vs. left

Tricuspid heart valve and tri-lobed lung both on the right side.
Bicuspid and bi-lobed lung both on the left side.

Thoracic duct: relation to azygous vein and esophagus

"The **duck** between **2 gooses**":
Thoracic **duct** (duck) is between 2 gooses, azy**gous** and esopha**gus**.

Maxillary artery branches

"**DAM I AM P**iss **D**runk **B**ut **S**tupid **D**runk **I**Prefer, **M**ust **P**hone
Alcoholics **A**nonymous":
Deep auricular
Anterior tympanic
Middle meningeal
Inferior alveolar
Accessory meningeal
Masseteric
Pterygoid
Deep temporal
Buccal
Sphenopalatine
Descending palatine

Abdominal muscles

"Spare **TIRE** around their abdomen":
Transversus abdominis
Internal abdominal oblique
Rectus abdominis
External abdominal oblique

Anterior forearm muscles: superficial group

"Pimps F*ck Prostitutes ForFun":

Pronator teres
Flexor carpi radialis
Palmaris longous
Flexor carpi ulnaris
Flexor digitorum superficialis

Bicipital groove: attachments of muscles near it

"The lady between two majors":

Teres major attaches to medial lip of groove.
Pectoralis major to lateral lip of groove.
Latissimus (Lady) is on floor of groove, between the 2 majors.

Brachioradialis: function, innervation, one relation, one attachment

BrachioRadialis:

Function: Its the Beer Raising muscle, flexes elbow, strongest when wrist is oriented like holding a beer.
Innervation: Breaks Rule: it's a flexor muscle, But Radial. (Radial nerve usually is for extensors: Recall BEST rule: B was for brachioradialis).
Important relation: Behind it is the Radial nerve in the cubital fossa.
Attachment: Attaches to Bottom of Radius.

Elbow: muscles that flex it

Three B's Bend the elBow:
Brachialis
Biceps
Brachioradialis

Elbow: which side has common flexor origin
FM (as in FM Radio):
Flexor **M**edial, so Common Flexor Origin is on the medial side

Erector spinae muscles
"**IL**ove **S**ex":
   From lateral to medial:
Iliocostalis
Longissimus
Spinalis
   Alternatively: "**IL**ong for **S**pinach"
   "Sex" helps you think of "Erector", but "Long" and "Spinach" help
   you remember the muscles' names.

Eye rotation by oblique muscles
"**IL**ove **S&M**":
Inferior oblique: **L**ateral eye rotation.
Superior oblique: **M**edial eye rotation.

Interossei muscles: actions of dorsal vs. palmar in hand
"**PAd** and **DAb**":
The **P**almar **Ad**duct and the **D**orsal **Ab**duct.
Use your **hand** to **dab** with a **pad**.

Intrinsic muscles of hand (palmar surface)
"**A OF A OF A**":
   Thenar, lateral to medial:
Abductor pollicis longus
Opponens pollicis
Flexor pollicis brevis
Adductor pollicis.
   Hypothenar, lateral to medial:
Opponens digiti minimi

Flexor digiti minimi
Abductor digiti minimi

Inversion vs. eversion muscles in leg

Second letter rule for inversion/eversion:
Eversion muscles:
pErineus longus
pErineus brevis
pErineus terius
Inversion muscles:
tIbialis anterior
tIbialis posterior

Lumbricals action

Lumbrical action is to hold a pea, that is to flex the metacarpophalangeal joint and extend the interphalangeal joints. When look at hand in this position, can see this makes an "L" shape, since **L** is for Lumbrical.

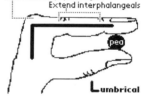

Muscles: potentially absent ones

Muscles which may be absent but may be important:
5 P's:
Palmaris longus [upper limb]
Plantaris [lower limb]
Peroneus tertius [lower limb]
Pyramidalis [anterior abdominal wall]
Psoas minor [posterior abdominal wall]

Oblique muscles: direction of externals vs. internals

"Hands in your pockets":

When put hands in your pockets, fingers now lie on top of external obliques and fingers point their direction of fibers: down and towards midline.

Note: "oblique" tells that must be going at an angle.

Internal obliques are at right angles to external

Plantarflexion vs. dorsiflexion

Plantar flexion occurs when you squish a **Plant** with your foot.

Popliteal fossa: muscles arrangement

The two Semi's go together, Semimembranosus and Semitendonosus.

The **M**embranosus is **M**edial and since the two semis go together, Semitendonosus is also medial.

Therefore, Biceps Femoris has to be lateral.

Of the semi's, to remember which one is superficial: the **T**endonosus is on **T**op.

Pterygoid muscles: function of lateral vs. medial

"Look at how your jaw ends up when saying first syllable of '**La**teral' or '**Me**dial' ":

"**La**": your jaw is now **open**, so **La**teral **opens** mouth.

"**Me**": your jaw is still **closed**, so **me**dial **closes** the mandible

Rotator cuff muscles

"The **SITS** muscles":

Clockwise from top:

Supraspinatus

Infraspinatus

Teres **minor**

Subscapularis

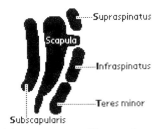

A pro baseball pitcher has injured his rotator cuff muscles. As a result, he **SITS** out for the rest of thegame, and then gets sent to the **minor** leagues.

Serratus anterior: innervation
SALT:
Serratus Anterior = Long Thoracic.

Serratus anterior: innervation and action
"C5-6-7raise your arms up to heaven":
Long thoracic nerve roots (567) innervate Serratus anterior.
Test C567 roots clinically by ability to raise arm past 90 degrees.

Soleus vs. gastrocnemius muscle function
"Stand on your Soles. Explosive gas":
You stand on soles of your shoes, so Soleus is for posture.
Gasoline is explosive, so Gastrocnemius is for explosive movement.

Supination vs. pronation
"SOUPination": Supination is to turn your arm palm up, as if you are holding a bowl of soup.
"POUR-nation": Pronation is to turn your arm with the palm down, as if you are pouring out whatever is your bowl.
   Alternatively, Pronation donation: Pronation is palm facing downward, as if making a donation.

Bell's palsy: symptoms
BELL'S Palsy:
Blink reflex abnormal
Earache
Lacrimation [deficient, excess]
Loss of taste
Sudden onset
Palsy of VII nerve muscles
   All symptoms are unilateral.

Brachial plexus branches

"**M**y **A**unt **R**aped **M**y **U**ncle":
From lateral to medial:
Musculocutaneous
Axillary
Radial
Median
Ulnar

Brachial plexus subunits

"**R**andy **T**ravis **D**rinks **C**old **B**eer":
Roots
Trunks
Divisions
Cords
Branches
Alternatively: "**R**ead **T**he**D**amn **C**adaver **B**ook!"
Alternatively: "**R**eal **T**exans **D**rink **C**oors **B**eer

Brachial plexus: branches of posterior cord

STAR:
Subscapular [upper and lower]
Thoracodorsal
Axillary
Radial

Buttock quadrant safest for needle insertion

"Shut **up** and **buttout**":
The **Up**per **Out**er quadrant of the **Butt**ock safely avoids hitting
sciatic nerve.

Carpal tunnel syndrome causes

MEDIAN TRAP:

Myxoedema

Edema premenstrually

Diabetes

Idiopathic

Agromegaly

Neoplasm

Trauma

Rheumatoid arthritis

Amyloidosis

Pregnancy

Mnemonic fits nicely since median nerve is trapped.

Cervical plexus: arrangement of the important nerves

"**GLAST**":

4 compass points: clockwise from north on the right side of neck:

Great auricular

Lesser occipital

Accessory nerve pops out between L and S

Supraclavicular

Transverse cervical

See diagram.

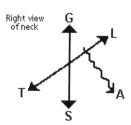

Deep tendon reflexes: root supply

God designed body reflexes according to a nursery rhyme:

One, two-- buckle my shoe. **Three, four**-- kick the door.**Five, six**-- pick up sticks.**Seven, eight**-- shut the gate.

S1,2 = ankle jerk

L3,4 = knee jerk

C5,6 = biceps and brachioradialis

C7,8 = triceps

Diaphragm innervation

"**3, 4, 5** keeps the diaphragm alive":
Diaphragm innervation is cervical roots **3**, **4**, and **5**.

Extraocular muscles cranial nerve innervation

"**LR6SO4 rest 3**":
Lateral **R**ectus is **6**th
Superior **O**blique is **4**th
rest are all **3**rd cranial nerve

Facial nerve: branches after Stylomastoid foramen

"**T**en **Z**ulus **B**uggered **M**y **C**at (**P**ainfully)":
From superior to inferior:
Temporal branch
Zygomatic branch
Buccal branch
Mandibular branch
Cervical branch
(**P**osterior auricular nerve)

Temporal
Zygomatic
Buccal
Mandibular
Posterior
Auricular
Cervical

Alternatively: "**PA**ssing **T**hrough **Z**anzibar **B**y**M**otor **C**ar" (**PA** for Posterior Auricular).

Lingual nerve course

The Lingual nerve
Took a curve
Around the Hyoglossus.
"Well I'll be f*#ked!"
Said Wharton's Duct,
"The bastard's gone and crossed us!"

Lumbar plexus

"**I, IG**et **L**aid **O**n **F**ridays":
Iliohypogastric [L1]
Ilioinguinal [L1]
Genitofemoral [L1, L2]
Lateral femoral cutaneous [L2, L3]
Obtruator [L2, L3, L4]
Femoral [L2, L3, L4]

> Alternatively: "**I** twice **G**et**L**aid **O**n **F**ridays".
> Alternatively: "**I**nterested **I**n **G**etting **L**aid **O**n **F**ridays?"

Lumbar plexus roots

"**2 from 1, 2 from 2, 2 from 3**":
2 nerves from **1** root: Ilioinguinal (L1), Iliohypogastric (L1).
2 nerves from **2** roots: Genitofemoral (L1,L2), Lateral Femoral (L2,L3).
2 nerves from **3** roots: Obturator (L2,L3,L4), Femoral (L2,L3,L4).

Median nerve: hand muscles innervated

"The **LOAF** muscles":
Lumbricals 1 and 2
Opponens pollicis
Abductor pollicis brevis
Flexor pollicis brevis

> Alternatively: **LLOAF**, with 2 L's, to recall there's 2 lumbricals.
> To remember that these are the **Me**dian nerve muscles, think "**Me**at **LOAF**".

Median nerve: recognizing it in an opened axilla

The Median nerve is the Middle of a giant capital "**M**" formed by the musculocutaneous and ulnar nerves.

Pectoral nerves: path of lateral vs. medial

"Lateral Less, Medial More":

Lateral pectoral nerve only goes through Pectoralis major, but
Medial pectoral nerve goes though both Pectoralis major and minor.

Pelvis: sacral innervation

"S2,3,4 keeps the 3 P's off the floor (Penis, Poo, and Pee).
  S2,3,4 innervates the anal sphincter, urethral sphicter, and causes
  erection.

Penis autonomic innervation actions

"Parasympathetic Puts it up. Sympathetic Spurts it out".
Alternatively: "Point and Shoot": Parasympathetic Points it,
Sympathetic Shoots out the semen.
  Erection and Ejaculation (Emission).

Radial nerve: muscles innervated

"Try ABig Chocolate Chip Sundae, Double Dip Cherries And
Peanuts Preferably Included":
  In order of their innervation, proximal to distal:
Triceps
Anconeus
Brachioradialis
ext. Carpi radialis longus
ext. Carpi radialis brevis
Supinator
ext. Digitorum
ext.Digiti minimi
ext. Carpi ulnaris
Abductor poll.longus
ext. Poll. brevis
ext. P poll. longus

ext. Indicis

For the neighboring words that start with the same letter (eg: chocolate and chip), notice that the **longer** word in the mnemonic, corresponds to the longer of the two muscle names (ex: ext. carpi radialis **longus** and ext. carpi radialis brevis)

Radial nerve: muscles supplied (simplified)

"**BEST** muscles":

Brachioradialis
Extensors
Supinator
Triceps

Scalp: nerve supply

GLASS:

Greater occipital/ **G**reater auricular
Lesser occipital
Auriculotemporal
Supratrochlear
Supraorbital

Spinal cord: length in vertebral column

SCULL:

Spinal **C**ord **U**nti**LL**2 (LL).

Thigh: innervation by compartment

"**MAP OF Sciatic**":

Medial compartment: **O**bturator
Anterior compartment: **F**emoral
Posterior compartment: **Sciatic**

So all the thigh muscles in that compartment get innervated by that nerve.

Trigeminal nerve: where branches exit skull

"**S**tanding **R**oom **O**nly":
Superior orbital fissure is V1
foramen**R**otundum is V2
foramen**O**vale is V3

V3 innervated muscles (branchial arch 1 derivatives)

"**M.D. My TV**":
Mastication [masseter, temporalis, pterygoids]
Digastric [anterior belly]
Mylohyoid
tensor**T**ympani
tensor**V**eli palatini

V3: sensory branches

"**Bucca**neers **Are Inferior Lingu**ists":
Buccal
Auriculotemporal
Inferior alveolar
Lingual

Vagus nerve: path into thorax

"I **Left** my **Aunt** in **Vegas**":
Left Vagus nerve goes **Ant**erior descending into the thorax.

Anatomical planes: coronal, horizontal, sagittal

Coronal: A classic painting/stained glass window of a saint/angel has a **corona** radiating around the
person's head. The plane of the glass/page is cutting their head in the coronal plane.
Horizontal: Someone coming over the **horizon** has their abdomen

cut in the horizontal plane.
Sagittal: the remaining one by default.

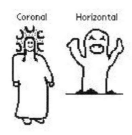

Coronal   Horizontal

Cubital fossa contents

"Really Need Booze To Be At My Nicest":
From lateral to medial:
Radial Nerve
Biceps Tendon
Brachial Artery
Median Nerve

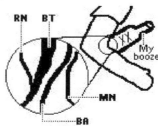

Hand: nerve lesions

DR CUMA:
Drop=Radial nerve
Claw=Ulnar nerve
Median nerve=Ape hand (or Apostol [preacher] hand)

Inguinal canal: walls

"MALT: 2M, 2A, 2L, 2T":
Starting from superior, moving around in order to posterior:
Superior wall (roof): 2 Muscles:
internal oblique Muscle
transverse abdominus Muscle
Anterior wall: 2 Aponeuroses:
Aponeurosis of external oblique
Aponeurosis of internal oblique
Lower wall (floor): 2 Ligaments:

inguinalLigament
lacunarLigament
Posterior wall: 2**T**s:
Transversalis fascia
conjoint**T**endon

Mediastinums: posterior mediastinum structures
There are 4 birds:
The esopha**GOOSE** (esophagus)
The va**GOOSE** nerve
The azy**GOOSE** vein
The thoracic **DUCK** (duct)

Perineal vs. peroneal
Peri**n**eal is **in** between the legs.
Per**on**eal is **on** the leg.

Retroperitoneal structures list
SAD PUCKER:
Suprarenal glands
Aorta & IVC
Duodenum (half)
Pancreas
Ureters
Colon (ascending & descending)
Kidneys
Esophagus (anterior & left covered)
Rectum

Superior mediastinum contents

"**BATS&TENT**":

Brachiocephalic veins

Arch of aorta

Thymus

Superior vena cava

Trachea

Esophagus

Nerves (vagus & phrenic)

Thoracic duct

Superior mediastinum: contents

PVT Left BATTLE:

Phrenic nerve

Vagus nerve

Thoracic duct

Left recurrent laryngeal nerve (not the right)

Brachiocephalic veins

Aortic arch (and its 3 branches)

Thymus

Trachea

Lymph nodes

Esophagus

Supine vs. prone body position

"**Supine** is on your **spine**.

Therefore, prone's the "other" one.

Also, **prone** to suffocate in **prone** position.

Bronchi: which is more vertical

"**Right** on **Red**":

Many places allow making a **right** hand turn at a **red** light, if you first come to a complete **stop**.

A child swallowing a **red** penny is more likely to get it **stop**ped down the **right** bronchus, since it is more vertical.

Bronchopulmonary segments of right lung

"**A PALM** Seed **M**akes **A**nother **L**ittle **P**alm":

In order from superior to inferior:

Apical
Posterior
Anterior
Lateral
Medial
Superior
Medial basal
Anterior basal
Lateral basal
Posterior basal

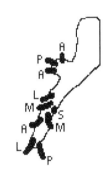

Lung lobes: one having lingula, lobe numbers

Lingula is on **L**eft.

The lingula is like an atrophied lobe, so the left lung must have 2 "other" lobes, and therefore right lung has 3 lobes.

Nasal cavity components

"**N**ever **C**all **M**e **N**eedle **N**ose!"

Nares [external]
Conchae
Meatuses
Nares [internal]
Nasopharynx

Note mnemonic sentence is nasally-related.

Pleura surface markings

"All the even ribs, in order: **2,4,6,8,10,12** show its route":

Rib**2**: sharp angle inferiorly
Rib**4**: the left pleura does a lateral shift to accommodate heart
Rib**6**: both diverge laterally
Rib**8**: midclavicular line
Rib**10**: midaxillary line
Rib**12**: the back
    See diagram.

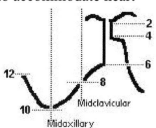

Tonsils: The three types

"**PPL** (people) have tonsils":

Pharyngeal
Palatine
Lingual

Voicebox: names of parts in sagittal cross-section

"There's 3 **V**'s in your Voicebox":

Vestibular fold
Ventricle
Vocal fold

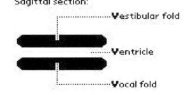

Note: Vestibular and Vocal cord also known as false and true cords respectively.

Anteflexed vs. anteverted: what bodypart each describes

"**Ante**flexed and **Ante**verted both bend toward **Ante**rior".
The "V" words go together: Verted is for the cerVix (therefore flexed must be uterus).

Broad ligament: contents

BROAD:

Bundle (ovarian neurovascular bundle)
Round ligament

Ovarian ligament
Artefacts (vestigial structures)
Duct (oviduct)

Scrotum layers

"**S**ome **D**amn **E**nglishman **C**alled **I**t **T**he **Testis**":
   From superficial to deep:
Skin
Dartos
External spermatic fascia
Cremaster
Internal spermatic fascia
Tunica vaginalis
Testis

Sperm pathway through male reproductive tract

SEVEN UP:
Seminiferous tubules
Epididymis
Vas deferens
Ejaculatory duct
Nothing
Urethra
Penis

Sperm: path through male reproductive system

"My boyfriend's name is **STEVE**":
Seminiferous **T**ubules
Epididymis
Vas deferens
Ejaculatory duct

Spermatic cord contents
"**P**iles **D**on't **C**ontribute **T**o **AG**ood **S**ex **L**ife":
Pampiniform plexus
Ductus deferens
Cremasteric artery
Testicular artery
Artery of the ductus deferens
Genital branch of the genitofemoral nerve
Sympathetic nerve fibers
Lymphatic vessels

Arm fractures: nerves affected by humerus fracture location
ARM fracture:
  From superior to inferior:
Axillary: head of humerus
Radial: mid shaft
Median: supracondular

Carpal bones
"**S**top **L**etting **T**hose **P**eople **T**ouch **T**he **C**adaver's **H**and":
  Proximal row, lateral-to-medial:
Scaphoid
Lunate
Triquetrum
Pisiform
  Distal row, lateral-to-medial:
Trapezium
Trapezoid
Capitate
Hamate

Carpal bones: trapezium vs. trapezoid location

Since there's two T's in carpal bone mnemonic sentences, need to know which T is where:

Trapezi**UM** is by the th**UMB**, Trapezi**OID** is in**SIDE**.

Alternatively, Trapezi**UM** is by the th**UMB**, Trapez**OID** is by its **SIDE**.

Carpel bones

"**S**o **L**ong **T**o **P**inky, **H**ere **C**omes **T**he **T**humb":

Proximal row, lateral-to-medial, then distal row, medial-to-medial:

Scaphoid

Lunate

Triquetrium

Pisiform

Hamate

Capate

Trapezoid

Trapezium

Cartilage derivatives of 1st pharyngeal arch (mandibular)

"**I'MAS**uper **S**exy **G**uy" (or Girl):

Incus

Malleus

Anterior ligament of malleus

Spine of sphenoid

Sphenomandibular ligament

Genial tubercle of mandible

Cranial bones
"**PEST OF** 6":

Parietal

Ethmoid

Sphenoid

Temporal

Occipital

Frontal

The 6 just reminds that there's 6 of them to remember.

Foramen ovale contents
OVALE:

Otic ganglion (just inferior)

V3 cranial nerve

Accessory meningeal artery

Lesser petrosal nerve

Emissary veins

Genu valgum vs. genu vargum
Genu val**GUM** (knock-knee): knees are **GUM**med together.

Varum (bowleg) is the other by default, or **Far** rhymes with **Var**, so knees are **far** apart.

Hand fractures: Colle's vs. Smith's
Colle's fracture: arm in fall position makes a 'C' shape.

Smith's fracture: arm in fall position makes a 'S' shape.

See diagram.

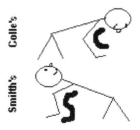

Joints in the midline

"**SC**":

In medial line, below **S**econd **C**ervical, joints are **S**econdary **C**artilaginous and usually have a di**SC.**

Notes: secondary cartilaginous is also known as symphysis. The one that doesn't have a disc is xiphi-sternal.

Lordosis vs. kyphosis

Lordosis: **L**umbar.

KYphosis is **HY** up on the spine.

Medial malleolus: order of tendons, artery, nerve behind it

"**T**om, **D**ick, **A**nd**N**ervous **H**arry":

From anterior to posterior:

Tibialis

Digitorum

Artery

Nerve

Hallicus

Full names for these are: Tibialis Posterior, Flexor Digitorum Longus, Posterior Tibial Artery, Posterior Tibial Nerve, Flexor Hallicus Longus.

Alternatively: "**T**om, **D**ick **AN**d**H**arry".

Alternatively: "**T**om, **D**ick **A**nd**N**ot **H**arry".

Navicular contacts 3 of 5 cuneiform bones

"**Nav**icular is like the **Nav**igator logo":

There are 3 things coming off each.

See diagram.

Therefore, cuboid has to contact 2 of the 5.

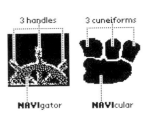

3 handles   3 cuneiforms

NAVIgator   **NAVI**cular

Ossification ages
"Every Potential Anatomist Should Know When"
When they ossify, in order of increasing year:
Elbow: **16** years
Pelvis, Ankle: **17** years
Shoulder, Knee: **18** years
Wrist: **19** years

Rib costal groove: order of intercostal blood vessels and nerve
VAN:
From superior to inferior:
Vein
Artery
Nerve

Superior orbital fissure: structures passing through
"Lazy French Tarts Lie Naked In Anticipation Of Sex":
Lacrimal nerve
Frontal nerve
Trochlear nerve
Lateral nerve
Nasociliary nerve
Internal nerve
Abducens nerve
Ophthalmic veins
Sympathetic nerves

Tibia: muscles of pes anserinus (the muscles attached to tibia's medial side)
"A Girl between Two Sargeants":
Gracilus is **between**
Sartorius and
Semitendonosus

Vertebrae: recognizing a thoracic from lumbar

Examine vertebral body shape:

Thoracic is **heart**-shaped body since your **heart** is in your **thorax**.

Lumbar is **kidney-bean** shaped since **kidneys** are in **lumbar** area.
See diagram.

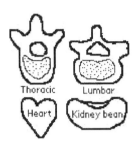

Wrist: radial side vs. ulnar side

Make a fist with your thumb up in the air and say "**Rad!**".

Your thumb is now pointing to your **Rad**ius.

Note: 'Rad!' was a late 80's catchphrase, short for 'Radical'. Things that were good were called 'Rad'.

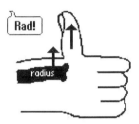

Xylocaine: where not to use with epinephrine

"Nose, Hose, Fingers and Toes"

Vasoconstrictive effects of xylocaine with epinephrine are helpful in providing hemostasis while suturing. However, may cause local ischemic necrosis in distal structures such as the digits, tip of nose, penis, ears.

Spinal anesthesia agents

"Little **B**oys **P**refer **T**oys":

Lidocaine

Bupivicaine

Procaine

Tetracaine

Knowledge Level 3, System: Nervous

Anonymous Contributor

Anesthesia machine/room check

MS MAID:

Monitors (EKG, SpO2, EtCO2, etc)

Suction

Machine check (according to ASA guidelines)

Airway equipment (ETT, laryngoscope, oral/nasal airway)

IV equipment

Drugs (emergency, inductions, NMBs, etc)

General anaesthesia: equipment check prior to inducing

MALES:

Masks

Airways

Laryngoscopes

Endotracheal tubes

Suction/ Stylette, bougie

Endotracheal intubation: diagnosis of poor bilateral breath sounds after intubation

DOPE:

Displaced (usually right mainstem, pyreform fossa, etc.)

Obstruction (kinked or bitten tube, mucuous plug, etc.)

Pneumothorax (collapsed lung)

Esophagus

BEHAVIOURAL SCIENCE / PSYCHOLOGY

Cluster personality disorders

Cluster **A** Disorder = **A**typical. Unusual and eccentric.

Cluster **B** Disorder = **B**east. Uncontrolled wildness.

Cluster **C** Disorder = **C**oward [avoidant type], **C**ompulsive [obsessive-compulsive type], or **C**lingy [dependent type].

Depression: major episode characteristics

SPACE DIGS:

Sleep disruption

Psychomotor retardation

Appetite change

Concentration loss

Energy loss

Depressed mood

Interest wanes

Guilt

Suicidal tendencies

Gain: primary vs. secondary vs. tertiary

Primary: **P**atient's **P**syche improved.

Secondary: **S**ymptom **S**ympathy for patient.

Tertiary: **T**herapist's gain.

Middle adolescence (14-17 years): characteristics

HERO:

Heterosexual crushes/ **H**omosexual Experience

Education regarding short term benefits

Risk taking

Omnipotence

And there is interest in being a Hero (popular).

Narcolepsy: symptoms, epidemiology

CHAP:

Cataplexy

Hallucinations

Attacks of sleep

Paralysis on waking

Usual presentation is a young male, hence "chap".

Sleep stages: features

DElta waves during **DE**epest sleep (stages 3 & 4, slow-wave).

d**REa**M during **REM** sleep.

Keober-Ross dying process: stages

"**D**eath **A**lways **B**rings **G**reat **A**cceptance":

Denial

Anger

Bargaining

Grieving

Acceptance

Impotence causes

PLANE:

Psychogenic: performance anxiety

Libido: decreased with androgen deficiency, drugs

Autonomic neuropathy: impede blood flow redirection

Nitric oxide deficiency: impaired synthesis, decreased blood pressure

Erectile reserve: can't maintain an erection

Male erectile dysfunction (MED): biological causes

MED:

Medicines(propranalol, methyldopa, SSRI, etc.)

Ethanol

Diabetes mellitus

Premature ejaculation: treatment

2 S's:

SSRIs [eg: fluoxitime]

Squeezing technique [glans pressure before climax]

More detail with 2 more S's:

Sensate-focus excercises [relieves anxiety]

Stop and start method [5-6 rehearsals of stopping stimulation before climax]

B vitamin names

"The **R**hythm **N**early **P**roved **C**ontagious":
  In increasing order:
Thiamine (B1)
Riboflavin (B2)
Niacin (B3)
Pyridoxine (B6)
Cobalamin (B12)
Knowledge Level 2, System: Alimentary
Anonymous Contributor

Essential amino acids

"**PVT. TIM HALL** always **arg**ues, never **ti**res":
Phe
Val
Thr
Trp
Ile
Met
His
Arg
Lue
Lys

  Always argues: the A is for Arg, not Asp.
  'Never tires': T is not Tyr, but is both Thr and Trp.

Fasting state: branched-chain amino acids used by skeletal muscles

"Muscles **LIV**e fast":

Leucine
Isoleucine
Valine

Folate deficiency: causes

A FOLIC DROP:

Alcoholism
Folic acid antagonists
Oral contraceptives
Low dietary intake
Infection with Giardia
Celiac sprue
Dilatin
Relative folate deficiency
Old
Pregnant

Glycogen storage: Anderson's (IV) vs. Cori's (III) enzyme defect

ABCD:

Anderson's=**B**ranching enzyme.
Cori's=**D**ebranching enzyme.
Otherwise, can't really distinguish clinically.

Glycogen storage: names of types I through VI

"**V**iagra **P**ills **C**ause **AM**ajor **H**ardon":

Von Gierke's
Pompe's
Cori's
Anderson's
McArdle's
Her's

Glycolysis steps

"Goodness Gracious, Father Franklin **DidGo ByP**icking Pumpkins (to) **Prepare Pie**s":

Glucose
Glucose-6-P
Fructose-6-P
Fructose-1,6-diP
Dihydroxyacetone-P
Glyceraldehyde-P
1,3-**Bi**phosphoglycerate
3-**P**hosphoglycerate
2-**P**hosphoglycerate (to)
Phosphoenolpyruvate [**PEP**]
Pyruvate

'Did', 'By' and 'Pies' tell you the first part of those three: di-, bi-, and py-.

'PrEPare' tells location of PEP in the process.

Hypervitaminosis A: signs and symptoms

"Increased Vitamin A makes you **HARD**":

Headache/ **H**epatomegaly
Anorexia/ **A**lopecia
Really painful bones
Dry skin/ **D**rowsiness

Infantile Beriberi symptoms

Restlessness
Sleeplessness
Breathlessness
Soundlessness (aphonia)
Eatlessness (anorexia)
Great heartedness (dilated heart)

Alternatively: Get 5 of 'em with **BERI**: **B**reathless/ **B**ig hearted, **E**atless, **R**estless, **I**nsomnia.

Phosphorylation cascade: action during low glucose

"In the Phasted State, Phosphorylate":
The phosphorylation cascade becomes active when blood glucose is low.

Type 1 glycogen storage disease

Type **1** = one (**Von**), ie Von Giereke's disease

Van den Bergh reaction (Jaundice test)

"**I**ndirect reacting bilirubin = **U**nconjugated bilirubin":
Both start with vowels, so they go together: **I**ndirect &**U**nconjugated.

Vitamin B3 (niacin, nicotinic acid) deficiency: pellagra

The 3 **D**'s of pellagra:
Dermatitis
Diarrhea
Dementia
  Note vitamin B**3** is the **3** D's.

Vitamins: which are fat soluble

KADE: (SHIV **KHEDA**)
Vitamin **K**
Vitamin **A**
Vitamin **D**
Vitamin **E**

Coagulation common pathway: factors in order

10 + 5 - 2 = 13
Coagulation common pathway:
Factor **X** to Factor **V** to Factor **II** to Factor **XIII**

Fabry's disease

FABRY'S:

Foam cells found in glomeruli and tubules/ **F**ebrile episodes
Alpha galactosidase A deficiency/ **A**ngiokeratomas
Burning pain in extremities/ **B**UN increased in serum/ **B**oys
Renal failure
YX genotype (male, X linked recessive)
Sphingolipidoses

Hemoglobin binding curve: causes of shift to right

"**CADET**, face **right!**":

CO2
Acid
2,3-**D**PG (aka 2,3 BPG)
Exercise
Temperature

Porphyrias: acute intermittent porphyria symptoms

5 P's:

Pain in abdomen
Polyneuropathy
Psychologial abnormalities
Pink urine
Precipitated by drugs (eg barbiturates, oral contraceptives, sulpha drugs)

Sickle cell disease pathophysiology

SICKle cell disease is due to a **S**ubstitution of the **SICK**sth amino acid of the B chain.

Vitamin K dependent cofactors

"**Seve**ral **Ten**d **ToNi**cely **S**top **C**lots":

Factor **Seve**n, **Ten**, **Two**, **Ni**ne.

Protein **S**, Protein **C**.

Adrenaline mechanism

"**ABC** of Adrenaline":

Adrenaline--> activates **B**eta receptors--> increases **C**yclic AMP

Insulin: function

INsul**IN** stimulates **2** things to go

IN2 cells: Potassium and Glucose.

BUN:creatinine elevation: causes

ABCD:

Azotremia (pre-renal)

Bleeding (GI)

Catabolic status

Diet (high protein parenteral nutrition)

G6PD: oxidant drugs inducing hemolytic anemia

AAA:

Antibiotic (eg: sufamethoxazole)

Antimalarial (eg: primaquine)

Antipyretics (eg: acetanilid, but not aspirin or acetaminophen)

Carbon monoxide: electron transport chain target

"CO blocks CO":

Carbon monoxide (CO) blocks Cytochrome Oxidase (CO)

Citric acid cycle compounds

"Can IKeep Selling Sex For Money, Officer?":

Citrate
Isocitrate
alphaKetogluterate
Succinyl CoA
Succinate
Fumerate
Malate
Oxaloacetate

DNA bond strength (nucleotides)

"Crazy Glue":

Strongest bonds are between Cytosine and Guanine, strong like
Crazy Glue (3 H-bonds), whereas the A=T only have 2 H-bonds.
  This is relevant to DNA replication, as the weaker A=T will be the
  site where RNA primer makes the initial break.

Electron transport chain: Rotenone's site of action

Rotenone is a site specific inhibitor of complex one.

Enzyme kinetics: competitive vs. non-competitive inhibition

With Kompetitive inhibition: Km increases; no change in Vmax.
With Non-kompetitive inhibition: No change in Km; Vmax
decreases.

Enzymes: classification

"Over The HILL":

Oxidoreductases
Transferases
Hydrolases
Isomerases
Ligases
Lyases

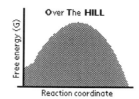

Enzymes get reaction over the hill. See diagram.

Enzymes: competitive inhibitors
"**Competition** is hard because we have to travel **more kilometers (Km)** with the **same velocity**":
With **competitive** inhibitors, **velocity remains same** but **Km increases**

G protein type for respective receptors
"**KISS** and **KICK** till you're **SICK** of **SEX**" (QISS and QIQ till you're SIQ of SQS):
    This gives the G-protein type (**Gq**, **Gi**, or **Gs**) for all the receptors.
    Receptors are in alphabetical order:
alpha1=**Q**
alpha2=**I**
beta1=**S**
beta3=**S**
M1=**Q**
M2=**I**
M3=**Q**
D1=**S**
D2=**I**
H1=**Q**
H2=**S**
V1=**Q**
V2=**S**

Metabolism sites
"Use **both** arms to **HUG**":
Heme synthesis
Urea cycle
Gluconeogenesis
These reactions occur in **both** cytoplasm and mitochondria

Na/K pump: concentrations of Na vs. K on inside/outside of cell, pump action, number of molecules moved

HIKIN':

There is a **HI**gh K concentration **IN**side the cell.

From this can deduce that the Na/K pump pumps K into cell and Na out of cell.

Alternatively: When I was learning this pump (circa 1992), a band that was "**in**" was **K**ris **K**ross, and a band that was "**out**" was "Sha **Na Na Na**":

So pump moves **K K** (2 K) **in** and **Na Na Na** (3 Na) out.

Sadly, as infectious as their debut album was, Kris Kross can really no longer be classed as "in".

Na+/K+ pump: movement of ions and quantity

K+ and **in** each consist of **2** characters, so so 2 K+ are pumped in.

Na+ and **out** each consist of **3** characters, so 3 Na+ are pumped out.

Phenylketonuria: which enzyme is deficient

PHenylketonuria is caused by a deficiency of:

Phenylalanine

Hydroxylase

Pompe's disease: type

"Police = Po + lys":

Pompe's disease is a **lys**osomal storage disease (alpha 1,4 glucosidase).

Pyruvate: products of complete oxidation

"**4** Naked **F**un **3** Coeds + **1** Guy":

Complete oxidation of pyruvate yields:

4 NADH

FADH2

3 CO2

1 GTP

Tangier's disease: hallmark

"**Tangier**ene tonsils":

Hallmark is large orange tonsils.

Important clinical note: there is **no** increased risk of atherosclerosis, just like eating tangerenes.

CARDIOLOGY

Aortic regurgitation: causes

CREAM:

Congenital

Rheumatic damage

Endocarditis

Aortic dissection/ Aortic root dilatation

Marfan's

Aortic stenosis characteristics

SAD:

Syncope

Angina

Dyspnoea

Apex beat: abnormalities found on palpation, causes of impalpable

HILT:

Heaving

Impalpable

Laterally displaced

Thrusting/ Tapping

If it is impalpable, causes are **COPD**:

COPD

Obesity

Pleural, Pericardial effusion

Dextrocardia

Apex beat: differential for impalpable apex beat
DOPES:

Dextrocardia

Obesity

Pericarditis/ Pericardial tamponade/ Pneumothorax

Emphysema

Sinus inversus/ Student incompetence/ Scoliosis/ Skeletal abnormalities (eg pectus excavatum)

Atrial fibrillation: causes
A S#!T:

Alcohol

Stenosis (mitral valve)

Hypertension

Infarction/ Ischaemia

Thyrotoxicosis

Atrial fibrillation: causes
PIRATES:

Pulmonary: PE, COPD

Iatrogenic

Rheumatic heart: mirtral regurgitation

Atherosclerotic: MI, CAD

Thyroid: hyperthyroid

Endocarditis

Sick sinus syndrome

Atrial fibrillation: management
ABCD:

Anti-coagulate

Beta-block to control rate

Cardiovert

Digoxin

Beck's triad (cardiac tamponade)

3 D's:

Distant heart sounds

Distended jugular veins

Decreased arterial pressure

Betablockers: cardioselective betablockers

"**B**etablockers **A**cting **E**xclusively **A**t **M**yocardium"

Cardioselective betablockers are:

Betaxolol

Acebutelol

Esmolol

Atenolol

Metoprolol

CHF: causes of exacerbation

FAILURE:

Forgot medication

Arrhythmia/ **A**naemia

Ischemia/ **I**nfarction/ **I**nfection

Lifestyle: taken too much salt

Upregulation of CO: pregnancy, hyperthyroidism

Renal failure

Embolism: pulmonary

Coronary artery bypass graft: indications

DUST:

Depressed ventricular function

Unstable angina

Stenosis of the left main stem

Triple vessel disease

Coronary artery bypass graft: indications
DUST:

Depressed ventricular function
Unstable angina
Stenosis of the left main stem
Triple vessel disease

Depressed ST-segment: causes
DEPRESSED ST:

Drooping valve (MVP)
Enlargement of LV with strain
Potassium loss (hypokalemia)
Reciprocal ST- depression (in I/W AMI)
Embolism in lungs (pulmonary embolism)
Subendocardial ischemia
Subendocardial infarct
Encephalon haemorrhage (intracranial haemorrhage)
Dilated cardiomyopathy
Shock
Toxicity of digitalis, quinidine

ECG: left vs. right bundle block
"**WiLLiaMMaRRoW**":

W pattern in V1-V2 and **M** pattern in V3-V6 is **L**eft bundle block.
M pattern in V1-V2 and **W** in V3-V6 is **R**ight bundle block.
Note: consider bundle branch blocks when QRS complex is wide.

Exercise ramp ECG: contraindications
RAMP:

Recent MI
Aortic stenosis
MI in the last 7 days
Pulmonary hypertension

Heart compensatory mechanisms that 'save' organ blood flow during shock

"Heart **SAVER**":

Symphatoadrenal system
Atrial natriuretic factor
Vasopressin
Endogenous digitalis-like factor
Renin-angiotensin-aldosterone system
   In all 5, system is activated/factor is released

JVP: wave form

ASK ME:

Atrial contraction
Systole (ventricular contraction)
Klosure (closure) of tricusps, so atrial filling
Maximal atrial filling
Emptying of atrium
   See diagram.

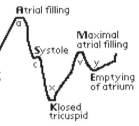

MI: basic management

BOOMAR:

Bed rest
Oxygen
Opiate
Monitor
Anticoagulate
Reduce clot size

MI: signs and symptoms
PULSE:

Persistent chest pains
Upset stomach
Lightheadedness
Shortness of breath
Excessive sweatin

MI: therapeutic treatment
"O BATMAN!":

Oxygen
Beta blocker
ASA
Thrombolytics (eg heparin)
Morphine
Ace prn
Nitroglycerin

MI: therapeutic treatment
MONAH:

Morphine
Oxygen
Nitrogen
Aspirin
Heparin

MI: treatment of acute MI
COAG:

Cyclomorph
Oxygen
Aspirin
Glycerol trinitrate

Mitral stenosis (MS) vs. regurgitation (MR): epidemiology

MS is a female title (**Ms.**) and it is female predominant.
MR is a male title (**Mr.**) and it is male predominant.

Murmur attributes

"**IL PQRST**" (person has ill PQRST heart waves):
Intensity
Location
Pitch
Quality
Radiation
Shape
Timing

Murmurs: innocent murmur features

8 S's:
Soft
Systolic
Short
Sounds (S1 & S2) normal
Symptomless
Special tests normal (X-ray, EKG)
Standing/ Sitting (vary with position)
Sternal depression

Murmurs: louder with inspiration vs expiration

LEft sided murmurs louder with **E**xpiration
RIght sided murmurs louder with **I**nspiration.

Murmurs: questions to ask

SCRIPT:

Site

Character (eg harsh, soft, blowing)

Radiation

Intensity

Pitch

Timing

Murmurs: right vs. left loudness

"**RILE**":

Right sided heart murmurs are louder on **I**nspiration.

Left sided heart murmurs are loudest on **E**xpiration.

Murmurs: systolic vs. diastolic

PASS: **P**ulmonic &**A**ortic **S**tenosis=**S**ystolic.

PAID: **P**ulmonic &**A**ortic **I**nsufficiency=**D**iastolic.

Myocardial infarctions: treatment

INFARCTIONS:

IV access

Narcotic analgesics (eg morphine, pethidine)

Facilities for defibrillation (DF)

Aspirin/ **A**nticoagulant (heparin)

Rest

Converting enzyme inhibitor

Thrombolysis

IV beta blocker

Oxygen 60%

Nitrates

Stool Softeners

Pericarditis: causes
CARDIAC RIND:
Collagen vascular disease
Aortic aneurysm
Radiation
Drugs (such as hydralazine)
Infections
Acute renal failure
Cardiac infarction
Rheumatic fever
Injury
Neoplasms
Dressler's syndrome

Pericarditis: EKG
"PericarditiS":
PR depression in precordial leads.
ST elevation.

Peripheral vascular insufficiency: inspection criteria
SICVD:
Symmetry of leg musculature
Integrity of skin
Color of toenails
Varicose veins
Distribution of hair

Pulseless electrical activity: causes
PATCH MED:
Pulmonary embolus
Acidosis
Tension pneumothorax
Cardiac tamponade

Hypokalemia/ Hyperkalemia/ Hypoxia/ Hypothermia/ Hypovolemia
Myocardial infarction
Electrolyte derangements
Drugs

Rheumatic fever: Revised Jones' criteria

JONES crITERIA:

Major criteria:

Joint (arthritis)

Obvious (Cardiac)

Nodule (Rheumatic)

Erythema marginatum

Sydenham chorea

Minor criteria:

Inflammatory cells (leukocytosis)

Temperature (fever)

ESR/CRP elevated

Raised PR interval

Itself (previous Hx of Rheumatic fever)

Arthralgia

ST elevation causes in ECG

ELEVATION:

Electrolytes

LBBB

Early repolarization

Ventricular hypertrophy

Aneurysm

Treatment (eg pericardiocentesis)

Injury (AMI, contusion)

Osborne waves (hypothermia)

Non-occlusive vasospasm

Supraventricular tachycardia: treatment

ABCDE:

Adenosine

Beta-blocker

Calcium channel antagonist

Digoxin

Excitation (vagal stimulation)

Ventricular tachycardia: treatment

LAMB:

Lidocaine

Amiodarone

Mexiltene/ **M**agnesium

Beta-blocker

CHEMISTRY

Benzene ring: order of substituents

"Benzene likes to **ROMP**": (**OM P**RAKASH)

From R group moving around the ring:

R group

Ortho

Meta

Para

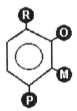

Cation vs. anion: positive vs. negative

The **t** in cation looks like a plus sign: "ca+ion".

Cation is positive, anion is negative.

Cis/trans (geometric) isomer nomenclature

"**Z**ame **Z**ide. **E**pposite.":

Z is the 2 functional groups on the same side of double bond.

E is for opposite sides.

Cis/trans (geometric) isomers: arrangement of functional groups

Cis starts with a **C** and the functional groups form a **C**.
Trans, therefore is the other one by default.

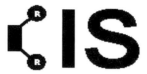

Gibb's free energy formula

"Good Honey Tastes Sweet":
$(delta)\mathbf{G} = \mathbf{H} - \mathbf{T}(delta)\mathbf{S}$

Oxidation vs. reduction: electrochemical cell and electron gain/loss

AN OIL RIG CAT:
At the **AN**ode, **O**xidation **I**nvolves **L**oss of electrons.
Reduction **I**nvolves **G**aining electrons at the **CAT**hode.

DERMATOLOGY

Clubbing: causes

CLUBBING:
Cyanotic heart disease
Lung disease (hypoxia, lung cancer, bronchiectasis, cystic fibrosis)
UC/Crohn's disease
Biliary cirrhosis
Birth defect (harmless)
Infective endocarditis
Neoplasm (esp. Hodgkins)
GI malabsorption

White patch of skin: differential
"**Vitiligo PATCH**":
Vitiligo
Pityriasis alba/ Post-inflammatory hypopigmentation
Age related hypopigmentation
Tinea versicolor/ Tuberous sclerosis (ashleaf macule)
Congenital birthmark
Hansen's (leprosy)

Wound healing: factors delaying
DID NOT HEAL:
Drugs
Infection/ Icterus/ Ischemia
Diabetes
Nutrition
Oxygen (hypoxia)
Toxins
Hypothermia/ Hyperthermia
EtOH
Acidosis
Local anesthetics

Branchial arch giving rise to aorta
"**Aor**- from **Four**":
Aorta is from fourth arch.

Tetrology of Fallot
"Don't **DROP** the baby":
Defect (VSD)
Right ventricular hypertrophy
Overriding aorta
Pulmonary stenosis

Potter syndrome: features
POTTER:
Pulmonary hypoplasia
Oligohydrominios
Twisted skin (wrinkly skin)
Twisted face (Potter facies)
Extremities defects
Renal agenesis (bilateral)

Cranial and spinal neural crest: major derivatives
GAMES:
Glial cells (of peripheral ganglia)
Arachnoid (and pia)
Melanocytes
Enteric ganglia
Schwann cells

Neuroectoderm derivatives

Neuroectoderm gives rise to:

Neurons

Neuroglia

Neurohypophysis

piNeurol (pineal) gland

Fetal alcohol syndrome (FAS): features

FAS:

Facial hypoplasia/ Forebrain malformation

Attention defecit disorder/ Altered joints

Short stature/ Septal defects/ Small I.Q

Mesoderm components

MESODERM:

Mesothelium (peritoneal, pleural, pericardial)/ Muscle (striated, smooth, cardiac)

Embryologic

Spleen/ Soft tissue/ Serous linings/ Sarcoma/ Somite

Osseous tissue/ Outer layer of suprarenal gland (cortex)/ Ovaries

Dura/ Ducts of genitalia

Endothelium

Renal

Microglia/ Mesenchyme/ Male gonad

Teratogenesis: when it occurs

TEratogenesis is most likely during organogenesis--between the:

Third and

Eighth weeks of gestation.

Weeks 2, 3, 4 of development: an event for each
Week **Two**: **Bi**laminar germ disc.
Week **Three**: **Tri**laminar germ disc.
Week **Four**: **Four** limbs appear.

Placenta-crossing substances
"**WANTM**y **H**ot **D**og":
Wastes
Antibodies
Nutrients
Teratogens
Microorganisms
Hormones/ **HIV**
Drugs

EMERGENCY MEDICINE

Ipecac: contraindications
4 C's:
Comatose
Convulsing
Corrosive
hydro**C**arbon

Acute LVF management
LMNOP:
Lasex (frusemide)
Morphine (diamorphine)
Nitrates
Oxygen (sit patient up)
Pulmonary ventilation (if doing badly)

Atrial fibrillation: causes of new onset
THE ATRIAL FIBS:

Thyroid

Hypothermia

Embolism (P.E.)

Alcohol

Trauma (cardiac contusion)

Recent surgery (post CABG)

Ischemia

Atrial enlargement

Lone or idiopathic

Fever, anemia, high-output states

Infarct

Bad valves (mitral stenosis)

Stimulants (cocaine, theo, amphet, caffeine)

JVP: raised JVP differential
PQRST (EKG waves):

Pericardial effusion

Quantity of fluid raised (fluid over load)

Right heart failure

Superior vena caval obstruction

Tricuspid stenosis/ Tricuspid regurgitation/ Tamponade (cardiac)

MI: immediate treatment
DOGASH:

Diamorphine

Oxygen

GTN spray

Asprin 300mg

Streptokinase

Heparin

PEA/Asystole (ACLS): etiology
ITCHPAD:

Infarction

Tension pneumothorax

Cardiac tamponade

Hypovolemia/ Hypothermia/ Hypo-, Hyperkalemia/ Hypomagnesmia/ Hypoxemia

Pulmonary embolism

Acidosis

Drug overdose

Shock: signs and symptoms
TV SPARC CUBE:

Thirst

Vomiting

Sweating

Pulse weak

Anxious

Respirations shallow/rapid

Cool

Cyanotic

Unconscious

BP low

Eyes blank

Subarachnoid hemorrhage (SAH) causes
BATS:

Berry aneurysm

Arteriovenous malformation/ Adult polycystic kidney disease

Trauma (eg being struck with baseball **bat**)

Stroke

Syncope causes, by system

HEAD HEART VESSELS:

CNS causes include HEAD:

Hypoxia/ **H**ypoglycemia

Epilepsy

Anxiety

Dysfunctional brain stem (basivertebral TIA)

Cardiac causes are HEART:

Heart attack

Embolism (PE)

Aortic obstruction (IHSS, AS or myxoma)

Rhythm disturbance, ventricular

Tachycardia

Vascular causes are VESSELS:

Vasovagal

Ectopic (reminds one of hypovolemia)

Situational

Subclavian steal

ENT (glossopharyngeal neuralgia)

Low systemic vascular resistance (Addison's, diabetic vascular neuropathy)

Sensitive carotid sinus

Ventricular fibrillation: treatment

"Shock, Shock, Shock, Everybody Shock, Little Shock, Big Shock, Momma Shock, Poppa Shock":

Shock= Defibrillate

Everybody= Epinephine

Little= Lidocaine

Big= Bretylium

Momma= MgSO4

Poppa= Pocainamide

Vfib/Vtach drugs used according to ACLS

"Every Little Boy Must Pray":

Epinephrine
Lidocaine
Bretylium
Magsulfate
Procainamide

Diabetic ketoacidosis management

F*¢KING:

Fluids (crytalloids)
Urea (check it)
Creatinine (check it)/ Catheterize
K+ (potassium)
Insulin (5u/hour. Note: sliding scale no longer recommended in the UK)
Nasogastic tube (if patient comatose)
Glucose (once serum levels drop to 12)

Coma causes checklist

AEIOU TIPS:

Acidosis/ Alcohol
Epilepsy
Infection
Overdosed
Uremia
Trauma to head
Insulin: too little or or too much
Pyschosis episode
Stroke occurred

Meningicoccal meningitis: complications

SAD REP:

Sepsis/ **S**hock/ **S**ubdural effusion

Ataxia/ **A**bscess (brain)

DIC/ **D**eafness

Retardation

Epilepsy

Paralysis

Miosis: causes of pin-point pupils

CPR ON SLIME:

Clonidine

Phenothiazines

Resting (deep sleep)

Opiates

Narcotics

Stroke (pontine hemorrhage)

Lomotil (diphenoxylate)

Insecticides

Mushrooms/ **M**uscarinic (inocybe, clitocybe)

Eye drops

Neurological focal deficits

10 S's:

Sugar (hypo, hyper)

Stroke

Seizure (Todd's paralysis)

Subdural hematoma

Subarachnoid hemorrhage

Space occupying lesion (tumor, avm, aneurysm, abscess)

Spinal cord syndromes

Somatoform (conversion reaction)

Sclerosis (MS)

Some migraines

Unconciousness: differential
FISH SHAPED:
Fainted
Illness/ Infantile febrile convulsions
Shock
Head injuries
Stroke (CVE)
Heart problems
Asphxia
Poisons
Epilepsy
Diabetes

Coma and signicantly reduced conscious state causes: causes
COMA:
CO_2 and CO excess
Overdose: TCAs, Benzos, EtOH, insulin, paracetamol, etc.
Metabolic: BSL, Na^+, K^+, Mg^{2+}, urea, ammonia, etc.
Apoplexy: stroke, SAH, extradural, subdural, Ca, meningitis, encephalitis, cerebral abscess, etc.

Malignant hyperthermia treatment
"Some Hot Dude Better Give Iced Fluids Fast!" (Hot dude = hypothermia):
Stop triggering agents
Hyperventilate/ Hundred percent oxygen
Dantrolene (2.5mg/kg)
Bicarbonate
Glucose and insulin
IV Fluids and cooling blanket
Fluid output monitoring/ Furosemide/ Fast heart [tachycardia]

RLQ pain: differential

APPENDICITIS:

Appendicitis/ **A**bscess

PID/ **P**eriod

Pancreatitis

Ectopic/ **E**ndometriosis

Neoplasia

Diverticulitis

Intussusception

Crohns Disease/ **C**yst (ovarian)

IBD

Torsion (ovary)

Irritable Bowel Syndrome

Stones

Shock: types

RN CHAMPS:

Respiratory

Neurogenic

Cardiogenic

Hemorrhagic

Anaphylactic

Metabolic

Psychogenic

Septic

Alternatively: "**MR. C.H. SNAP**", or "**NH CRAMPS**".

ARDS: diagnostic criteria

ARDS:

Acute onset

Ratio (PaO2/FiO2) less than 200

Diffuse infiltration

Swan-Ganz Wedge pressure less than 19 mmHg

Asthma: management of acute severe

"O S#!T":

Oxygen (high dose: >60%)
Salbutamol (5mg via oxygen-driven nebuliser)
Hydrocortisone (or prednisolone)
Ipratropium bromide (if life threatening)
Theophylline (or preferably aminophylline-if life threatening)

Fall: potential causes

I'VE FALLEN:
Illness
Vestibular
Environmental
Feet/ Footwear
Alcohol and drugs
Low blood pressure
Low O2 states
Ears/ Eyes
Neuropathy

ENT

Oralpharangeal cancers: aetiology

6 S's:
Smoking
Spicy food
Syphilis
Spirits [booze]
Sore tooth
Sepsis
Also bezel nuts.

Nasopharyngeal carcinoma: classic symptoms
NOSE:
Neck mass
Obstructed nasal passage
Serous otitis media externa
Epistaxis or discharge
Knowledge Level 3, System: Pulmonary
Anonymous Contributor

EPIDEMIOLOGY / BIOSTATISTICS

Alcohol withdrawal effects
"**S#IT**":
Shakes/ **S**eizures/ **S**weats/ **S**tomach pains (n/v)
Hallucinosis (auditory)
Increased vitals/ **I**nsomnia
Tremens (delirium tremens-the lethal part)

Suicide risk factors
SAD PERSONS:
Sex: male
Age: young, elderly
Depression
Previous suicide attempts
Ethanol and other drugs
Reality testing/ **R**ational thought (loss of)
Social support lacking
Organized suicide plan
No spouse
Sickness/ **S**tated future intent

Accuracy of test: sensitivity vs. specificity

seNsitivity of a test: related to the rate of false Negatives.
sPecificity of a test: related to the rate of false Positives.
   Alternatively written:
seNsitive: No Non-Negatives.
sPecific: Puny Psuedo-Positives.

Hill criteria for causality

" 'ClownsPursuing Epidemiology' Commonly Behind The Silly Samples":
Consistency
Plausibility
Experimentation
Biological gradient
Coherence
Temporality
Strength of association
Specificity

Incidence vs. prevalence

Incidence: Initiate Infection InInterval.
Prevalence: Population's Percentage Positive.

Informed consent: requirements, exceptions

"Sign this DOC before we can start":
Discussion
Obtain agreement
Coercion-free
   Exceptions to informed consent are WIPE:
Waiver
Incompetent
Privilege (therapeutic privilege)
Emergency

Prevention: primary vs. secondary vs. tertiary

Primary: Predisposing factors decreased.

Secondary: Severity decreased.

Tertiary: Therapy, Training.

Recall bias

REcall bias is a problem with
REtrospective studies and is based on ability to
REmember.

GASTROENTEROLOGY

Bilirubin: common causes for increased levels

"**HOT** Liver":

Hemolysis

Obstruction

Tumor

Liver disease

Celiac sprue gluten sensitive enteropathy: gluten-containing grains

BROW:

Barley

Rye

Oats

Wheat

Flattened intestinal villi of celiac sprue are smooth, like an
eye**brow**.

Charcot's triad (gallstones)

"**Char**ge a **FEE**":

Charcot's triad is:

Fever

Epigastric & RUQ pain

Emesis & nausea

Cholangitis features
CHOLANGITITS:

Charcot's triad/ Conjugated bilirubin increase

Hepatic abscesses/ Hepatic (intra/extra) bile ducts/ HLA B8, DR3

Obstruction

Leukocytosis

Alkaline phosphatase increase

Neoplasms

Gallstones

Inflammatory bowel disease (ulcerative colitis)

Transaminase increase

Infection

Sclerosing

Cirrhosis: causes of hepatic cirrhosis
HEPATIC:

Hemochromatosis (primary)

Enzyme deficiency (alpha-1-anti-trypsin)

Post hepatic (infection + drug induced)

Alcoholic

Tyrosinosis

Indian childhood (galactosemia)

Cardiac/ Cholestatic (biliary)/ Cancer/ Copper (Wilson's)

Crohn's disease: morphology, symptoms
CHRISTMAS:

Cobblestones

High temperature

Reduced lumen

Intestinal fistulae

Skip lesions

Transmural (all layers, may ulcerate)

Malabsorption

Abdominal pain

Submucosal fibrosis

Digestive disorders: pH level

With **vomiting** both the pH and food come **up**.
With **diarrhea** both the pH and food go **down**.

GIT symptoms

BAD ANAL S#!T:

Bleeding

Abdominal pain

Dysphagia

Abdominal bloating

Nausea & vomiting

Anorexia/ **A**ppetite changes

Lethargy

S#!ts (diarrhea)

Heartburn

Increased bilirubin (jaundice)

Temperature (fever)

H. Pylori treatment regimen (rough guidelines)

"Please Make Tummy Better":

Proton pump inhibitor

Metronidazole

Tetracycline

Bismuth

   Alternatively: **TOMB**:

Tetracycline

Omeprazole

Metronidazole

Bismuth

Hepatic encephalopathy: precipitating factors

HEPATICS:

Hemorrhage in GIT/ Hyperkalemia
Excess protein in diet
Paracentesis
Acidosis/ Anemia
Trauma
Infection
Colon surgery
Sedatives

IBD: extraintestinal manifestations

A PIE SAC:

Aphthous ulcers
Pyoderma gangrenosum
Iritis
Erythema nodosum
Sclerosing cholangitis
Arthritis
Clubbing of fingertips

IBD: surgery indications

"I CHOP":

Infection
Carcinoma
Haemorrhage
Obstruction
Perforation
    "Chop" convenient since surgery chops them open.

Liver failure (chronic): signs found on the arms

CLAPS:

Clubbing

Leukonychia

Asterixis

Palmar erythema

Scratch marks

Pancreatitis (acute): causes

GET SMASHED:

Gallstones

Ethanol

Trauma

Steroids

Mumps

Autoimmune (PAN)

Scorpion stings

Hyperlipidemia/ Hypercalcemia

ERCP

Drugs (including azathioprine and diuretics)

Note: 'Get Smashed' is slang in some countries for drinking, and ethanol is an important pancreatitis cause.

Pancreatitis: criteria

PANCREAS:

PaO2 below 8

Age >55

Neutrophils: WCC >15

Calcium below 2

Renal: Urea >16

Enzymes: LDH >600; AST >200

Albumin below 32

Sugar: Glucose >10 (unless diabetic patient)

Pancreatitis: Ranson criteria for pancreatitis at admission
LEGAL:

Leukocytes > 16.000

Enzyme AST > 250

Glucose > 200

Age > 55

LDH > 350

Ulcerative colitis: complications
"**PAST** Colitis":

Pyoderma gangrenosum

Ankylosing spondylitis

Sclerosing pericholangitis

Toxic megacolon

Colon carcinoma

Vomiting: extra GI differential
VOMITING:

Vestibular disturbance/ Vagal (reflex pain)

Opiates

Migrane/ Metabolic (DKA, gastroparesis, hypercalcemia)

Infections

Toxicity (cytotoxic, digitalis toxicity)

Increased ICP, Ingested alcohol

Neurogenic, psychogenic

Gestation

Haemachromatosis complications
"HaemoChromatosis Can Cause Deposits Anywhere":

Hypogonadism

Cancer (hepatocellular)

Cirrhosis

Cardiomyopathy
Diabetes mellitus
Arthropathy

Diabetic ketoacidosis: precipitating factors

5 I's:
Infection
Ischaemia (cardiac, mesenteric)
Infarction
Ignorance (poor control)
Intoxication (alcohol)

GENETICS

Achrondroplasia dwarfism: inheritance pattern

Achondroplasia Dwarfism is Autosomal Dominant.

DiGeorge/ Velocardiofacial syndrome: features

CATCH 22:
Cardiac abnormalities
Abnormal facies
Thymic aplasia
Cleft palate
Hypocalcemia
22q11 deletion

Tay Sach's features

SACHS:
Spot in macula
Ashkenazic Jews
CNS degeneration
Hex A deficiency
Storage disease

Extra details with **TAY**:

Testing recommended

Autosomal recessive/ Amaurosis

Young death (<4 yrs)

Blots: function of Southern vs. Northern vs. Western

"SN0WDR0P":

Match up the 1st word letter with 2nd word letter:

Southern=**DNA**

Northern=**RNA**

Western=**Protein**

The 0's in snow drop are zeros, since there is no Eastern blot.

Cell cycle stages

"Go Sally Go! Make Children!":

G1 phase (Growth phase 1)

S phase (DNA Synthesis)

G2 phase (Growth phase 2)

M phase (Mitosis)

C phase (Cytokinesis)

Chromosome 15 diseases

Chromosome 15 has its own **MAP**:

Marfan syndrome

Angelman syndrome

Prader-Willi syndrome

Codons: nonsense mutation

"**Stop** talking **nonsense**!":

Nonsense mutation causes premature **stop**.

Cri-du-chat syndrome: chromosomal deletion causing it is 5p(-)

What's another name for a **cat** that's **five** letters long and starts with a **P**? (Answer: pussy).

Why is the cat **cry**ing? **Missing** its **P**.

DNA: Z vs. B form: which is inactive

ZZZZ is sleeping (inactive).

B form is therefore active DNA.

Down syndrome pathology

DOWN:

Decreased alpha-fetoprotein and unconjugated estriol (maternal)

One extra chromosome twenty-one

Women of advanced age

Nondisjunction during maternal meiosis

Exon vs. intron function

Exons **Ex**pressed.

InTrons **In Tr**ash.

Hurler syndrome features

HURLER'S:

Heptosplenomegaly

Ugly facies

Recessive (AR inheritance)

L-iduronidase deficiency (alpha)

Eyes clouded

Retarded

Short/ Stubby fingers

Imprinting diseases: Prader-Willi and Angelman

"**Pray** to an **Angel**":

Prader-Willi and **Angel**man are the 2 classic imprinting diseases.

Which disease results, depends on whether 15q deletion is maternal or paternal. Keep them straight by:

Paternal is Prader-Willi.

See diagram for cardinal symptom of each disease.

Marfan syndrome features

MARFAN'S:

Mitral valve prolapse

Aortic **A**neurysm

Retinal detachment

Fibrillin

Arachnodactyly

Negative **N**itroprusside test (differentiates from homocystinuria)

Subluxated lens

Nucleotides: class having the single ring

"Pyrimadines are **CUT** from purines"

Pyrimidines are:

Cytosine

Uracil

Thiamine

They are **cut** from purines so the pyrimadines must be smaller (one ring).

Nucleotides: double vs. triple bonded basepairs

"**TU** bonds" (two bonds):

T-A and **U**-A have**Two** bonds.

G-C therefore has the three bonds.

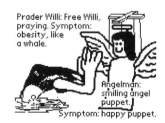

Prader Willi: Free Willi, praying. Symptom: obesity, like a whale.

Angelman: smiling angel puppet. Symptom: happy puppet.

Nucleotides: which are purines

"**Pure Silver**":

Chemical formula of **Pur**e silver is **Ag**.

Therefore, **Pur**ines are **A**denine and **G**uanine.

Pedigree symbols: gender and affected

Gender: The **cIR**cle is a **gIR**l [so boys are squares].

Affected: **Black plague** was a **disease**, so **black**-filled symbol means an **affected/diseased** person [so non-filled-in is unaffected].

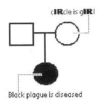

cIRcle is gIRl

Black plague is diseased

Taste buds: vallate vs. fungiform distribution

Cross sectional shape of the top of the bud tells their distribution.

Vallate: has a shallow 'V' at the top, so has a 'V' distribution at the back of the tongue.

Fungiform: top is **round** so it is towards the **round** end of the tongue. See diagram.

Note vallate is also sometimes called circumvallate.

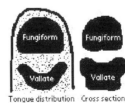

Fungiform   Fungiform

Vallate   Vallate

Tongue distribution   Cross section

Vascular endothelium: simplified cross-section
LIMA:
Lumen
Intima
Media
Adventitia

Leukocytes: granulated and agranulated
"**BEN**Loves **M**oney":
  Granulocytes:
Basophil
Eosinophil
Neurophil
  Agranulocytes:
Lymphocytes
Monocytes
  Alternatively: **Gran**pa **BEN**..." to keep the granulated group straight.

Mast cell primary granule contents
"**Mast**er, **His**Hepes Causes Choking &Gagging!":
Mast = **Mast** cell
His = **His**tamine
He= **He**parin
C = **C**hymase
Ch = **Ch**emotactic factor for eosinophils
Gag = **GAG**ase

Neutrophil's 2 distinctive physical features

1: There's up to **5 lobes** of the nucleus joined by thin appendages. Tie this to it being a neutrophil nucleus

by arranging the **5 lobes** into a **capital N for Neutrophil.**

2: the **chicken** leg (Barr Body) sticking out. Say it out loud: **chick-N**. The chick-**N** leg is for **N**eutrophil.

Neutrophil

chickeN leg

Muscle cells: cardiac vs. skeletal's nuclei location/number

Nuclei location mirrors where the muscle is located in human body. Heart muscle is in the **middle** of body, so heart muscle has nucleus in **middle**.

Skeletal muscles are at **periphery** of body, so nuclei are at **periphery**.

Also, you have 1 heart, so usually only 1 nucleus per heart muscle cell, but have many skeletal muscles,

so have many nuclei per long fibre.

See diagram.

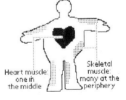

Heart muscle:
one in
the middle

Skeletal
muscle:
many at the
periphery

Muscle sarcomere: A vs. I as light or dark

There is only one vowel in "dark" and one vowel in "light".

These one vowels match up to their one letter names:

D**A**rk band is the **A** band.

L**I**ght band is the **I** band.

Muscle sarcomere: H line vs. Z disc location

HAZI (Hazy):

H line is in **A**-band.

Z disc is in the **I** band.

Graves disease: etiology

In **Graves** disease, the thyroid-stimulating immunoglobulins are of the Ig**G** class.

Lupus signs and symptoms

SOAP BRAIN:

Serositis [pleuritis, pericarditis]

Oral ulcers

Arthritis

Photosensitivity

Blood [all are low - anemia, leukopenia, thrombocytopenia]

Renal [protein]

ANA

Immunologic [DS DNA, etc.]

Neurologic [psych, seizures]

Celiac sprue features

CELIAC:

Cell-mediated autoimmune disease

European descent

Lymphocytes in Lamina propria/ Lymphoma risk

Intolerance of gluten (wheat)

Atrophy of villi in small intestine/ Abnormal D-xylose test

Childhood presentation

Atrophied villi cause less absorption, so diarrhea, weight loss, less energy.

Complement cascade initiating items: alternative vs. classic

Classic: Combined Complexes.

Alternative: Activators Alone, or IgA.

Complexes are made of Ab and Ag combined together.

Examples of activators: endotoxin, microbial surface.

Complement: function of C3a versus C3b

C3a: Activates Acute [inflammation].

C3b: Bonds Bacteria [to macrophages--easier digestion].

If wish to know more than just C3:

C3a, C4a, C5a activate acute.

C3b, C4b bind bacteria.

DiGeorge Syndrome: features

The disease of T's:

Third and 4th pharyngeal pouch absent.

Twenty-Two chromosome

T-cells absent

Tetany: hypocalcemia

Goodpasture's Syndrome components

GoodPasture is Glomerulonephritis and Pnuemonitits.

From autoantibodies attacking Glomerular and Pulmonary basement membranes.

Hypersensitivity reactions: Gell and Goombs nomenclature

ACID

From I to IV:

Anaphylactic type: type I

Cytotoxic type: type II

Immune complex disease: type III

Delayed hypersensitivity (cell mediated): type IV

Hypersensitivity: type IV example
Poison **IV**y causes type **IV** hypersensitivity.

Immunoglobulin (Ig) types: the important ones worth remembering, in order of appearance
MAGDElaine (a girl's name):

IgM

IgA

IgG

IgD

IgE

Magdelaine tells you the order they usually appear: **M** first, then **A or G**.

Alternatively: **IgM** is **IM**mediate.

Immunoglobulins, and order B cells present them
MADGE (character from the old dishwashing liquid commercial):

IgM

IgA

IgD

IgG

IgE

Order of presentation by B cells (which is made first, IgD or IgM?)B cells present **IgM** primarily, and then **IgD**.

Just remember why all of us are going through this pain...to become M.D's. For a B cell to be competent, it must get its **MD**.

Finally, by the same rule, B cells must first release **M** then **G** immunoglobulin on primary exposure.

Immunoglobulins: which crosses the placenta
Ig**G** crosses the placenta during **G**estation.

Interferon gamma: action on macrophages
"Th1nk BIG Mac Attack":
Th1 and NK cells Build Interferon Gamma.
Causes Macrophages to have an augmented Attack [by better lysosome function and increasing reactive oxygen metabolites, nitric oxide and defensins].

MHC I vs. MHC II properties
"Immunity helps to exterminate fun for bacteria"
See attached chart.

Cells with MHC class	Immune cells	All nucleated cells
T-cell MHC interaction	Helper T-cells	Cytotoxic T-cells
MHC name	Two (II)	One (I)
Exposed protein	External origin	Internal origin
1ST MHC use	Fungi	Viruses
CD type interaction	CD4+	CD8+
2ND MHC use	Bacteria	Cancer cells

Sjogren syndrome: morphology
"Jog through the MAPLES":
Sjogren is:
Mouth dry
Arthritis
Parotid enlarged
Lymphoma
Eyes dry
Sicca (primary) or Secondary
See diagram.

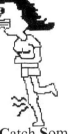

Sjogren Triad:
Dry eyes
Dry mouth
Arthritis

When you jog, you get dry eyes and mouth from wind, and sore joints from hitting the pavement.

T and B cells: types
When bacteria enter body, T-cell says to B: "Help Me Catch Some!"
B-cell replies: "My Pleasure!":
T-cell types:
Helper
Memory
Cytotoxic
Suppressor
B-cell types:
Memory cell
Plasma cell

ACEI: contraindictions
PARK:

Pregnancy

Allergy

Renal artery stenosis

K increase (hyperkalemia)

Anion gap metabolic acidosis: causes
A MUDPILE CAT:

Alcohol

Methanol

Uremia

Diabetic ketoacidosis

Paraldehyde

Iron/ Isoniazid

Lactic acidosis

Ethylene glycol

Carbamazepine

Aspirin

Toluene

Haematology: key numbers
3 and **4** are key in in haematology:

1.**34** cm3 of oxygen is carried by a gram of hemoglobin.

There's **3.4**mg of iron in each gram of hemoglobin.

There's an average of **3.4** lobes per neutrophil.

There's **34**mg bilirubin from each gram of hemoglobin.

Macrocytic anemia: causes

ABCDEF:

Alcohol + liver disease

B12 deficiency

Compensatory reticulocytosis (blood loss and hemolysis)

Drug (cytotoxic and AZT)/ **D**ysplasia (marrow problems)

Endocrine (hypothyroidism)

Folate deficieny/ **F**etus (pregnancy)

Metabolic acidosis: causes

KUSSMAL:

Ketoacidosis

Uraemia

Sepsis

Salicylates

Methanol

Alcohol

Lactic acidosis

Non-gap acidosis: causes

HARD UP:

Hyperalimentation

Acetazolamide (carbonic anhydrase inhibitors)

RTA

Diarrhea

Ureterosigmoidostomy

Pancreatic fistula

Pancytopaenia differential

"**A**ll **O**f **M**y **B**lood **H**as **T**aken **S**ome **P**oison":

Aplastic anaemias

Overwhelming sepsis

Megaloblastic anaemias

Bone marrow infiltration
Hypersplenism
TB
SLE
Paroxysmal nocturnal haemoglobinuria

Raynaud's disease: causes
BAD CT:
Blood disorders (eg polycythaemia)
Arterial (eg atherosclerosis, Buerger's)
Drugs (eg beta-blockers)
Connective tissue disorders (rheumatoid arthritis, SLE)
Traumatic (eg vibration injury)

Ulcers: types
VAN:
Venous/ Vasculitic
Arterial
Neuropathic

Acromegaly symptoms
ABCDEF:
Arthralgia/ Arthritis
Blood pressure raised
Carpal tunnel syndrome
Diabetes
Enlargemed organs
Field defect

Gynecomastia: common causes
GYNECOMASTIA:
Genetic Gender disorder (Klinefelter)
Young boy (pubertal)*
Neonate*
Estrogen
Cirrhosis/ Cimetidine/ Ca Channel blockers
Old age*
Marijuana
Alcoholism
Spironolactone
Tumors (Testicular & adrenal)
Isoniazid/ Inhibition of testosterone
Antineoplastics (Alkylating Agents)/ Antifungal(ketoconazole)
 * Asterisk indicates physiologic cause.

Hypercalcemia causes
MD PIMPS ME:
Malignancy
Diuretics (thiazide the main culprit)
Parathyroid (hyperparathyroidism)
Immobilization/ Idiopathic
Megadoses of vitamins A,D
Paget's disease
Sarcoidosis
Milk alkali syndrome
Endocrine (Addison's disease, thyrotoxicosis)

Hypercalcemia: causes
GRIM FED:
Granulomas (sarcoid, TB),
Renal faliure
Immobility (esp. long term)

Malignancy
Familial (eg familial hypocalciuric hypercalcemia)
Endocrine (see below for subtypes)
Drugs (esp. thiazide diuretics, lithium)
  Endocrine causes are **PATH**:
Phaeochromocytoma
Addison's disease
Thyrotoxicosis
Hyperparathyroidism

Hypercalcemia: differential
VITAMIN TRAPS:
Vitamin A and D intoxication
Immobilization
Thyrotoxicosis
Addison's disease/ Acidosis
Milk-alkali syndrome
Inflammatory disorders
Neoplastic disease
Thiazides, other drugs
Rhabdomyolysis
AIDS
Paget's disease/ Parenteral nutrition/ Parathyroid disease
Sarcoidosis

Pressure Sore: Norton Score
MAGIC:
Mobility
ADL
General condition
Incontinence
Conscious level

Pruritus without rash: DDx

ITCHING DX:

Infections (scabies, toxocariasis, etc)

Thyroidal and other endocrinopathies (eg diabetes mellitus)

Cancer

Hematologic diseases (eg iron deficiency)/ Hepatopathies/ HIV

Idiopathic

Neurotic

Gravid (pruritus of pregancy)

Drugs

eXcretory dysfunctions (eg uremia)

Rashes: time of appearance after fever onset

"**R**eally **S**ick **C**hildren **M**ust **T**ake **N**o **E**xercise":

Number of days after fever onset that a rash will appear:

1 Day: **R**ubella

2 Days: **S**carlet fever/ **S**mallpox

3 Days: **C**hickenpox

4 Days: **M**easles (and see the Koplik spots one day prior to rash)

5 Days: **T**yphus & rickettsia (this is variable)

6 Days: **N**othing

7 Days: **E**nteric fever (salmonella)

Alkalosis: metabolic changes in alkalosis

"Al-**K**-loss, Al-**Ca**-loss":

There is loss of **K**+ (hypokalemia) and **Ca**++ (hypocalcemia) in state of alkalosis.

Allopurinol: indications

STORE:

Stones (history of renal stones)

Tophaceous gout (chronic)

Over-producers of urate

Renal disease

Elderly

Bonus: Probenecid indications are basically the opposite of STORE (no renal stone history, etc.).

Dialysis indications

HAVE PEE:

Hyperkalemia (refractory)

Acidosis (refractory)

Volume overload

Elevated BUN (> 36 mM)

Pericarditis

Encephalopathy

Edema (pulmonary)

Renal failure (acute): management

Manage **AEIOU:**

Anemia/ Acidosis

Electrolyte and fluids

Infections

Other measures (eg nutrition, nausea, vomiting

Uremia

SIADH: causes

SIADH:

Surgery

Intracranial: infection, head injury, CVA

Alveolar: Ca, pus

Drugs: opiates, antiepileptics, cytotoxics, anti-psychotics

Hormonal: hypothyroid, low corticosteroid level

SIADH: diagnostic sign

Syndrome of **INAPP**ropriate Anti-Diuretic Hormone:

Increased

Na (sodium)

PP (urine)

SIADH is characterized by increased urinary sodium.

SIADH: major signs and symptoms

SIADH:

Spasms

Isn't any pitting edema (key DDx)

Anorexia

Disorientation (and other psychoses)

Hyponatremia

Eosinophilia: differential

NAACP:

Neoplasm

Allergy/ **A**sthma

Addison's disease

Collagen vascular diseases

Parasites

Polycythemia Rubra Vera (PRV): common symptoms

PRV:

Plethora/ **P**ruritis

Ringing in ears

Visual blurriness

SLE: factors that make SLE active

UV PRISM:

UV (sunshine)

Pregnancy

Reduced drug (eg steroid)
Infection
Stress
More drug

Splenomegaly: causes
CHICAGO:
Cancer
Hem, onc
Infection
Congestion (portal hypertension)
Autoimmune (RA, SLE)
Glycogen storage disorders
Other (amyloidosis)

Horner's syndrome: components
SAMPLE:
Sympathetic chain injury
Anhidrosis
Miosis
Ptosis
Loss of ciliospinal reflex
Enophthalmos

Lethargy, malaise causes
FATIGUED:
Fat/ Food (poor diet)
Anemia
Tumor
Infection (HIV, endocarditis)
General joint or liver disease
Uremia
Endocrine (Addison's, myxedema)
Diabetes/ Depression/ Drugs

Back pain causes

DISK MASS (since near vertebral disc):

Degeneration (DJD, osteoporosis, spondylosis)

Infection (UTI, PID, Pott's disease, osteomyelitis, prostatitis)/ **I**njury, fracture or compression fracture

Spondylitis (ankylosing spondyloarthropathies such as rheumatoid arthritis, Reiters, SLE)

Kidney (stones, infarction, infection)

Multiple myeloma/ **M**etastasis (from cancers of breast, kidney, lung, prostate, thyroid)

Abdominal pain (referred to the back)/ **A**neurysm

Skin (herpes zoster)/ **S**train/ **S**coliosis and lordosis

Slipped disk/ **S**pondylolisthesis

Behcet's syndrome: diagnostic criteria

PROSE:

Pathergy test (i/d saline injection)

Recurrent genital ulceration

Oral ulceration (recurrent)

Skin lesions

Eye lesions

Oral ulceration is central criteria, plus any 2 others.

ICU management: A to Z

A: Asepsis/ Airway

B: Bed sore/ encourage Breathing/ Blood pressure

C: Circulation/ encourage Coughing/ Consciousness

D: Drains

E: ECG

F: Fluid status

G: GI losses/ Gag reflex

H: Head positioning/ Height

I: Insensible losses

J: Jugular venous pulse

K: Kindness

L: Limb care/ Label

M: Mouth care

N: Nociception/ Nutrition

O: Oxygenation/ Orient the patient

P: Pulse/ Peristalsis/ Physiotherapy

Q: Quiet surroundings

R: Respiratory rate/ Restraint

S: Stress ulcer/ Suctioning

T: Temperature

U: Urine

V: Ventilator

W: Wounds/ Weight

X: Xerosis

Y: whY

Z: Zestful care of the patient

Left iliac fossa: causes of pain

SUPER CLOT:

Sigmoid diverticulitis

Uteric colic

PID

Ectopic pregnancy

Rectus sheath haematoma

Colorectal carcinoma

Left sided lower love pneumonia

Ovarian cyst (rupture, torture)

Threatened abortion/ Testicular torsion

Acute stridor: differential
ABCDEFGH:
With fever:
Abscess
Bacterial tracheitis
Croup
Diphtheria
Epiglottitis
Without fever:
Foreign body
Gas (Toxic Gas)
Hypersensitivity

Bronchiectasis: causes
A SICK AIRWAY:
Airway lesion, chronic obstruction
Sequestration
Infection, inflamation
Cystic fibrosis
Kartagners syndrome
Allergic brochopulmonary aspergilliosis
Immunodeficiencies (hypogammaglobinaemia, myeloma, lymphoma)
Reflux, inhalation injury
William Campbell syndrome (and other congenitals)
Aspiration
Yellow nail syndrome/ **Y**oung syndrome

Bronchiectasis: differential
BRONCHIECTASIS:
Bronchial cyst
Repeated gastric acid aspiration
Or due to foreign bodies

Necrotizing pneumonia
Chemical corrosive substances
Hypogammaglobulinemia
Immotile cilia syndrome
Eosinophilia (pulmonary)
Cystic fibrosis
Tuberculosis (primary)
Atopic bronchial asthma
Streptococcal pneumonia
In Young's syndrome
Staphylococcal pneumonia

Hemoptysis: causes
HEMOPTYSIS:
Haemorrhagic diathesis
Edema [LVF due to mitral stenosis]
Malignancy
Others [eg: vasculitis]
Pulmonary vascular abnormalities
Trauma
Your treatment [anticoagulants]
SLE
Infarction in lungs
Septic

Pleural effusion: investigations
PLEURA:
Pleural fluid (thoracentesis)
Lung, pleural biopsy
ESR
Ultrasound
Radiogram
Analysis of blood

Pulmonary edema: treatment

LMNOP:

Lasix

Morphine

Nitrates (NTG)

Oxygen

Position (upright vs. flat)

Pulmonary edema: treatments

MAD DOG:

Morphine

Aminophylline

Digitalis

Diuretics

Oxygen

GGases in blood (ABG's)

Pulmonary fibrosis: causes

SCAR:

Upper lobe:

Silicosis/ Sarcoidosis

Coal worker pneumonconiosis

Ankylosing spondylitis

Radiation

Lower lobe:

Systemic sclerosis

Cyptogenic fibrosing alveolitis

Asbetosis

Rheumatoid arthritis

Wheezing: causes

ASTHMA:

Asthma

Small airways disease

Tracheal obstruction
Heart failure
Mastocytosis or carcinoid
Anaphylaxis or allergy

Back trouble causes
O, VERSALIUS (Versalius was the name of a famous physician):
Osteomyelitis
Vertebral fracture
Extraspinal tumour
Spondylolisthesis
Ankylosing spondylitis
Lumbar disk increase
Intraspinal tumor
Unhappiness
Stress

INTERVIEWING / PHYSICAL EXAM

Abdomen assessment
To assess abdomen, palpate all 4 quadrants for **DR. GERM**:
Distension: liver problems, bowel obstruction
Rigidity (board like): bleeding
Guarding: muscular tension when touched
Eviseration/ Ecchymosis
Rebound tenderness: infection
Masses

Vomiting: non-GIT differential
ABCDEFGHI:
Acute renal failure
Brain [increased ICP]
Cardiac [inferior MI]

DKA

Ears [labyrinthitis]

Foreign substances [Tylenol, theo, etc.]

Glaucoma

Hyperemesis gravidarum

Infection [pyelonephritis, meningitis]

Heart valve auscultation sites

"**A**ll **P**atients **T**ake **M**eds":

Reading from top left:

Aortic

Pulmonary

Tricuspid

Mitral

See diagram.

Alternatively: **A**ll **P**rostitutes **T**ake **M**oney.

Alternatively: **AP**e **T**o **M**an.

Glasgow coma scale: components and numbers

Scale types is 3 **V**'s:

Visual response

Verbal response

Vibratory (motor) response

Scale scores are 4,5,6:

Scale of **4**: see so much **more**

Scale of **5**: talking **jive**

Scale of **6**: feels the **pricks** (if testing motor by pain withdrawl)

Mental state examination: stages in order

"**A**ssessed **M**ental **S**tate **T**o **B**e **P**ositively **C**linically **U**nremarkable":

Appearance and behaviour [observe state, clothing...]

Mood [recent spirit]

Speech [rate, form, content]

Thinking [thoughts, perceptions]
Behavioural abnormalities
Perception abnormalities
Cognition [time, place, age...]
Understanding of condition [ideas, expectations, concerns]

Pain history checklist

SOCRATES:

Site

Onset

Character

Radiation

Alleviating factors/ **A**ssociated symptoms

Timing (duration, frequency)

Exacerbating factors

Severity

Alternatively, **S**igns and **S**ymptoms with the 'S'.

Abdominal swelling causes

9 F's:

Fat

Feces

Fluid

Flatus

Fetus

Full-sized tumors

Full bladder

Fibroids

False pregnancy

Clinical examination: initial Inspection of patient from end of bed

ABC:

Appearance (SOB, pain, etc)

Behaviour

Connections (drips, inhalers, etc connected to patient)

Differential diagnosis checklist

"A VITAMIN C"

A and C stand for Acquired and Congenital

VITAMIN stands for:

Vascular

Inflammatory (Infectious and non-Infectious)

Trauma/ Toxins

Autoimmune

Metabolic

Idiopathic

Neoplastic

Example usage: List causes of decreased vision: Central retinal artery occlusion, Retinitis pigmentosa, Perforation to gobe, Chronic Gentamycin use, Ruematoid arthritis, Diabetes, Idiopathic, Any eye tumor, Myopia.

Differential diagnosis checklist

"I VINDICATE AID":

Idiopathic

Vascular

Infectious

Neoplastic

Degenerative

Inflammatory

Congenital

Autoimmune

Traumatic

Endocrinal and metabolic

Allergic

Iatrogenic

Drugs

Family history (FH)
BALD CHASM:

Blood pressure (high)
Arthritis
Lung disease
Diabetes
Cancer
Heart disease
Alcoholism
Stroke
Mental health disorders (depression, etc.)

Four point physical assessment of a disease
"**I**'m **AP**eople **P**erson":

Inspection
Auscultation
Percussion
Palpation

Medical history: disease checklist
MJ THREADS:

Myocardial infarction
Jaundice
Tuberculosis
Hypertension
Rheumatic fever/ **R**heumatoid arthritis
Epilepsy
Asthma
Diabetes
Strokes

Aside: "History" album was by Michael Jackson (MJ).

Past medical history (PMH)

VAMP THIS:

Vices (tobacco, alcohol, other drugs, sexual risks)

Allergies

Medications

Preexisting medical conditions

Trauma

Hospitalizations

Immunizations

Surgeries

Patient examination organization

SOAP:

Subjective: what the patient says.

Objective: what the examiner observes.

Assessment: what the examiner thinks is going on.

Plan: what they intend to do about it.

Patient profile (PP)

LADDERS:

Living situation/ Lifestyle

Anxiety

Depression

Daily activities (describe a typical day)

Environmental risks/ Exposure

Relationships

Support system/ Stress

Physical exam for 'lumps and bumps'

"6 Students and 3 Teachers go for **CAMPFIRE**":

Site, Size, Shape, Surface, Skin, Scar

Tenderness, Temperature, Transillumination

Consistency

Attachment
Mobility
Pulsation
Fluctuation
Irreducibility
Regional lymph nodes
Edge

Physical examination - correct order

"**IPalpateP**eople's Abdomens":
Inspection
Palpation
Percussion
Auscultation

Short statue causes

RETARD HEIGHT:
Rickets
Endocrine (cretinism, hypopituitarism, Cushing's)
Turner syndrome
Achondroplasia
Respiratory(suppurative lung disease)
Down syndrome
Hereditary
Environmental (postirradiation, postinfectious)
IUGR
GI (malabsorption)
Heart (congenital heart disease)
Tilted backbone (scoliosis)

Sign vs. symptom

s**I**gn: something **I** can detect even if patient is unconscious.
s**YM**ptom is something only h**YM** knows about.

Surgical sieve for diagnostic categories
INVESTIGATIONS:
Iatrogenic
Neoplastic
Vascular
Endocrine
Structural/ Mechanical
Traumatic
Inflammatory
Genetic/ Congenital
Autoimmune
Toxic
Infective
Old age/ Degenerative
Nutritional
Spontaneous/ Idiopathic

Breast history checklist
LMNOP:
Lump
Mammary changes
Nipple changes
Other symptoms
Patient risk factors

MICROBIOLOGY

E. coli: major subtypes, key point of each
"**HIT** by E. coli outbreak":
EnteroHemorrhagic:
HUS from **H**amburgers
EnteroInvasive:

Medical Mnemonics By FRK

Immune-mediated Inflammation
EnteroToxigenic:
Traveller's diarrhea

Entameoba histolytica: disease caused, action
EntAmoeba causes Amoebic dysEntery.
Action: histo (cell) lytic (burst), so it bursts cells.

Hepatitis: oral-fecal transmitted types
"A$$ Eaters":
Types A and E by oral-fecal route.

Vibrio: motility
"Vibrio Vibrates":
Vibrio is a genus of actively motile bacteria.

Endocarditis: indications for surgery
PUS RIVER:
Prosthetic valve endocarditis (most cases)
Uncontrolled infection
Supporative local complications with conduction abnormalities
Resection of mycotic aneurysm
Ineffective antimicrobial therapy (eg Vs fungi)
Valvular damage (significant)
Embolization (repeated systemic)
Refractory congestive heart failure

Endocarditis: lab results suggesting it
"High Tech Lab Results Point AtEndocarditis":
Hematuria
Thrombocytopenia
Leukocytosis, -penia
Red blood cell casta

Proteinuria

Anemia

Elevated ESR

Psedomonas aeruginosa: features

AERUGINOSA:

Aerobic

Exotoxin A

Rod/ **R**esistance

UTIs, burns, injuries

Green-blue dressings

Iron-containing lesions

Negative gram

Odor of grapes

Slime capsule sometimes (in CF pt)

Adherin pili

Acute post-streptococcal glomerulonephritis: classic presentation

"Sore **throat**, Face **bloat**, Pi$$ **coke**":

Sore **throat**: 1 week ago

Face **bloat**: facial edema

Pi$$ **coke**: coke-coloured urine

Alternatively, short version: "**Throat**, **bloat** and **coke**".

Proteus: disease caused

Firstly, "**PROT**eus hates **PROT**ons":

So what does it do to fight the protons? It has a urease that raises the pH.

Urea is in urine, so Proteus causes UTIs.

UTI-causing microorganisms

KEEPS:

Klebsiella

Enterococcus faecalis/ Enterobacter cloacae
E. coli
Pseudomonas aeroginosa/ Proteus mirabilis
Staphylococcus saprophyticcus/ Serratia marcescens

Endotoxin features
ENDOTOXIN:
Endothelial cells/ **E**dema
Negative (gram- bacteria)
DIC/ **D**eath
Outer membrane
TNF
O-antigen
X-tremely heat stable
IL-1
Nitric oxide/ **N**eutrophil chemotaxis

IgA protease-producing bacteria
"**Nice Strip** of **Ham**":
Neisseria
Streptococcus pneumonia
Haemophilus influenza

Meningitis: risk factors
"**C**an **I**nduce **S**evere **A**ttacks **Of**Head **PAINS**":
Cancer
Immunocompromised state
Sinusitis
Age extremes
Otitis
Head trauma
Parameningeal infection
Alcoholism

Infections (systemic, esp. respiratory)
Neurosurgical procedures
Splenectomy

Chlamydia: elementary vs. initial body location
Elementary: Extracellular
Initial: Intracellular

Common cold: viral causes
"Common cold (acute infectious rhinitis, coryza) is **PRIMA**rily caused by":
Paramyxoviruses
Rhinoviruses
Influenza viruses
Myxoviruses
Adenoviruses

DNA viruses: morphology rule of thumb
DNA:
Double-stranded
Nuclear replication
'**A**nhedral symmetry
Rule breakers: pox (cytoplasmic), parvo (single-stranded).

Gram+: bacterial cell wall
Gram+ has:
+hick pepidoglycan layer.
+eichoic acid in wall.

Neisseria: fermentation of N. gonorrhoeae vs. N. meningitidis
Gonorrhoeae: **G**lucose fermenter only.
Menin**G**itidis: **M**altose and **G**lucose fermenter.
Maltose fermentation is a useful property to know, since it's the classic test to distinguish the Neisseria types.

Obligate anaerobes: members worth knowing

ABC:
Actinomyces
Bacteroides
Clostridium

Picornavirus: features

PICORNAvirus:
Positive sense
ICOsahedral
RNA virus

RNA viruses: negative stranded

"**Ortho**dox **Rhab**bi's **Pa**rty **A**round**Fi**ne **Bun**nies":
Orthomyxo
Rhabdo
Paramyxo
Arena
Filo
Bunya

RNA viruses: positive stranded

"**Pico**Called **Flavi**o **To**Return **Re**nzo's **Corona**":
Picorna
Calici
Flavi
Toga
Retro
Reo
Corona

Staphylococcus aureus: diseases caused

SOFT PAINS:

Skin infections

Osteomyelitis

Food poisoning

Toxic shock syndrome

Pneumonia

Acute endocarditis

Infective arthritis

Necrotizing fasciitis

Sepsis

Streptococci: classification by hemolytic ability

Gamma: **Ga**rbage (no hemolytic activity).

Alpha: **Al**most (almost lyse, but incomplete).

Beta: **Be**st (complete lysis).

Streptococcus pyogenes: diseases caused

NIPPLES:

Necrotising fasciitis and myositis

Impetigo

Pharyngitis

Pneumonia

Lymphangitis

Erysipelas and cellulitis

Scarlet fever/ Streptococcal TSS

Streptococcus pyogenes: virulence factors

SMASHED:

Streptolysins

M protein

Anti-C5a peptidase

Streptokinase

Hyaluronidase

Exotoxin

DNAses

Urease positive organisms

PUNCH:

Proteus (leads to alkaline urine)

Ureaplasma (renal calculi)

Nocardia

Cryptoccocus (the fungus)

Helicobacter pylori

Influenza infection: clinical manifestations

"Having Flu Symptoms Can Make Moaning Children ANightmare":

Headache

Fever

Sore throat

Chills

Myalgias

Malaise

Cough

Anorexia

Nasal congestion

Klebsiella details

You tell the patient: "**Get UPS** you **fat alcoholic**":

UTI

Pneumonia

Sepsis

Fat capsule

Get up=**nonmotile** since no flagella.

Alcoholic=commonly seen in **alcoholic** and nosocomial patients.

Pneumonia: acute pneumonia infiltrates from different causes

"**P**yrogenic=**PMN**, **M**iscellaneous=**M**ononuclear":

Acute pneumonia caused by **P**yogenic bacteria: **PMN** infiltrate.

Acute pneumonia caused by **M**iscellaneous microbes: **M**ononuclear infiltrate.

Streptococci: Quellung reaction: positive sign, Strep type confirmed

"**Quell-lung**":

Quell: Capsules **swell** [+ve test].

Lung: S. **pnuemonia** [type confirmed].

You get **pneumonia** in your **lung**.

Gardnerella and Vaginalis vaginal infection diagnosis

"Take a **whiff** and get a **clue** for fishy bacteria":

Smells like fish (whiff test); clue cells seen under microscope.

Gardnerella= **G**ram negative.

Vaginalis= **V**ariable.

Teratogens: placenta-crossing organisms

ToRCHeS:

Toxoplasma

Rubella

CMV

Herpes simplex, **H**erpes zoster (varicella), **H**epatitis B,C,E

Syphilis

Alternatively: **TORCHES**: with **O**thers (parvo, listeria), add **HIV** to H's, **E**nteroviruses.

Trichomaniasis: features

5 F's:

Flagella

Frothy discharge

Fishy odor (sometimes)

Fornication (STD)
Flagyl (metronidazole) Rx

NEUROLOGY

Stroke risk factors
HEADS:
Hypertension/ **H**yperlipidemia
Elderly
Atrial fib
Diabetes mellitus/ **D**rugs (cocaine)
Smoking/ **S**ex (male)

Chorea: common causes
St. VITUS'S DANCE:
Sydenhams
Vascular
Increased RBC's (polycythemia)
Toxins: CO, Mg, Hg
Uremia
SLE
Senile chorea
Drugs
APLA syndrome
Neurodegenerative conditions: HD, neuroacanthocytosis, DRPLA
Conception related: pregnancy, OCP's
Endocrine: hyperthyroidism, hypo-, hyperglycemia

Congenital myopathy: features
DREAMS:
Dominantly inherited, mostly
Reflexes decreased
Enzymes normal

Apathetic floppy baby
Milestones delayed
Skeletal abnormalities

Dementia: reversible dementia causes

DEMENTIA:

Drugs/ Depression
Elderly
Multi-infarct/ Medication
Environmental
Nutritional
Toxins
Ischemia
Alcohol

Dementia: some common causes

DEMENTIA:

Diabetes
Ethanol
Medication
Environmental (eg CO poisoning)
Nutritional
Trauma
Infection
Alzheimer's

Dementia: treatable causes

DEMENTIA:

Drug toxicity
Emotional (depression, anxiety, OCD, etc.)
Metabolic (electrolytes, liver dz, kidney dz, COPD)
Eyes/ Ears (peripheral sensory restrictions)
Nutrition (vitamin, iron deficiencies/ **N**PH [Normal Pressure

Hydrocephalus]
Tumors/ Trauma (including chronic subdural hematoma)
Infection (meningitis, encephalitis, pneumonia, syphilis)
Arteriosclerosis and other vascular disease

Encephalitis: differential
HE'S LATIN AMERICAN:
Herpesviridae
Enteroviridae (esp. Polio)
Slow viruses (esp. JC, prions)
Syphilis
Legionella/ Lyme disease/ Lymphocytic meningoencephalitis
Aspergillus
Toxoplasmosis
Intracranial pressure
Neisseria meningitidis
Arboviridae
Measles/ Mumps/ Mycobacterium tuberculosis/ Mucor
E. coli
Rabies/ Rubella
Idiopathic
Cryptococcus/ Candida
Abscess
Neoplasm/ Neurocysticercosis
  Neurocysticercosis should be assumed with recent Latin American
  immigrant patient unless proven otherwise.

Head trauma: rapid neuro exam
  12 P's:
Psychological (mental) status
Pupils: size, symmetry, reaction
Paired ocular movememts
Papilloedema

Pressure (BP, increased ICP)
Pulse and rate
Paralysis, Paresis
Pyramidal signs
Pin prick sensory response
Pee (incontinent)
Patellar relex (and others)
Ptosis
   Reevaluate patient every 8 hrs.

Neurofibromatosis: diagnostic criteria
ROLANDO:
Relative (1st degree)
Osseous fibromas
Lisch nodules in eyes
Axillary freckling
Neurofibromas
Dime size cafe au lait spots
Optic gliomas

Neuropathy: diagnosis confirmation
NEuropathy:
Nerve conduction velocity
Electromyography

Ocular bobbing vs. dipping
"Breakfast is **fast**, Dinner is slow, both go **down**":
Bobbing is **fast**.
Dipping is **slow**.
In both, the initial movement is **down**.

Peripheral neuropathies: differential

DANG THERAPIST:

Diabetes

Amyloid

Nutritional (eg B12 deficiency)

Guillain-Barre

Toxic (eg amiodarone)

Heriditary

Endocrine

Recurring (10% of G-B) **A**lcohol

Pb (lead)

Idiopathic

Sarcoid

Thyroid

Ramsay-Hunt syndrome: cause and common feature

"**R**amsay **H**unt":

Etiology:

Reactivated

Herpes zoster

Complication:

Reduced

Hearing

Status epilepticus: treatment

"**T**hank **G**oodness **A**ll **C**erebral **B**ursts **D**issipate":

Thiamine

Glucose

Ativan

Cerebyx

Barbiturate

Diprivan

Vertigo: differential

VOMITS:

Vestibulitis

Ototoxic drugs

Meniere's disease

Injury

Tumor

Spin (benign positional vertigo)

NEUROSCIENCES

Argyll-Robertson Pupil features

Argyll Robertson Pupil (ARP)

Read it from front to back: it is **ARP**, standing for **A**ccomodation **R**eflex **P**resent.

Read it from back to front: it is **PRA**, standing for **P**upillary **R**eflex **A**bsent.

Auditory pathway: mandatory stops

"**C**ome **I**n **M**y **B**aritone":

Cochlear nucleus

Inferior colliculus

Medial geniculate nucleus

Brodmann's 41 (cortex)

Basal ganglia: indirect vs. direct pathway

The **In**direct pathway **In**hibits.

Direct pathway is hence the excitatory one.

Branchial arches: cranial nerve innervation

In Sensory/Motor/Both mnemonic 'Some Say Marry Money **B**ut My **B**rother Says **B**ig **B**oobs Matter More', the **B**'s also give **B**rancial arch nerves in order:

But (CN 5): 1st arch

Brother (CN7): 2nd arch
Big (CN9): 3rd arch
Boobs (CN 10): 4th arch

Broca's vs. Wernick's area: effect of damage to speech center
"**Broca**": your speech machinery is **Brok**en.
Broca is wanting to speak, but articulation doesn't work, and very slow.
"**Wer-nick**": "**were**" and "**nick**" are both words of English language, but together they are nonsensical.
Wernick is having good articulation, but saying words that don't make sense together.

Cerebellar damage symptoms
VANISHeD:
Vertigo
Ataxia
Nystagmus
Intention tremor
Slurred speech
Hypotonic reflexes
Dysdiadochokinesia.

Cerebellar deep nuclei
"Ladies **D**emand **E**xceptional **G**enerosity **F**rom**M**en":
The 4 nuclei, from lateral to medial:
[Lateral]
Dentate
Emboliform
Globose
Fastigial
[Medial]

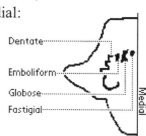

Cerebellar functional areas

Anatomical shape/location of cerebellar areas is a key to their function and related tract.

Vermis = **Spino**cerebellar = **Axial** equilibrium.

Vermis:right down the **axis** of cerebellum, and vertically segmented like a **spinal** column.

Flocculonodular lobe = **Vestibulo**cerebellar = **Ear**, eye, body coordination.

Flocculonodular lobe: flares out to the edges, just like **ears**.

Hemispheres of cerebellum = **Cerebro**cerebellar = **Peripheral** coordination.

Hemispheres: around **periphery** of cerebellum, and tract to **cerebral hemispheres**.

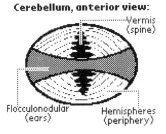

Cerebellum, anterior view:

Coronal section of brain: structures

"**InExtreme**Conditions **E**at **P**eople's **G**uts **In**stead of **T**heir **H**earts":
   From insula to midline:

Insula

Extreme capsule

Claustrum

External capsule

Putamen

Globis pallidus

Internal capsule

Thalamus

Hypothalamus

Cranial nerves

"On Old Olympus Towering Tops, AFinn And German Viewed Some Hops":

In order from 1 to 12:

Olfactory

Optic

Occulomotor

Trochlear

Trigeminal

Abducens

Facial

Auditory [or Vestibulocochlear]

Glossopharyngeal

Vagus

Accessory [or Spinal root of the accessory]

Hypoglossal

Alternatively:"Oh! Oh! Oh! To Touch And Feel AGirls Vagina, Ah! Heaven!".

Alternatively: "Oh, Oh, Oh, To Touch And Feel Virgin Girls Vaginas And Hymens".

Cranial nerves: olfactory and optic numbers

"You have **two eyes** and **one nose**":

Optic nerve is cranial nerve **two**.

Olfactory nerve is cranial nerve **one**.

Alternatively, note alphabetical order: oLfactory, and oPtic.

Cranial nerves: sensory, motor or both
"**S**ome **S**ay **M**arry **M**oney **B**ut **M**y **B**rother **S**ays **B**ig **B**rains **M**atter **M**ore":

From I to XII:

Sensory

Sensory

Motor

Motor

Both

Motor

Both

Sensory

Both

Both

Motor

Motor

Alternatives for "Brains": Boobs, Buns, Bras.

CSF circulation: function of choroid vs. arachnoid granules
Choroid **C**reates CSF.

Arachnoid granules **A**bsorb CSF.

Dysphagia vs. dysphasia
Dyspha**S**ia is for **S**peech

Dyspha**G**ia is for your **G**ut [swallowing].

GABA vs. Glu: the excitatory vs. inhibitory transmitter in brain (eg in basal ganglia)
When you **Glue** two things together, you add (+) those things together, therefore **Glu** is the excitatory one (+).

GABA is therefore the negative one.

Geniculate bodies: medial vs. lateral system
MALE:

Medial=**A**uditory. Lateral=**E**ye.

Medial geniculate body is for auditory system, lateral geniculate body is for visual system.

Can expand to **MALES** to remember Lateral=**E**ye=**S**uperior colliculus (thus medial is inferior colliculus by default).

Hypothalamus: feeding vs. satiety center
"Stim the **lat**, get **fat**":

Stimulating **lat**eral increases hunger.

"Stim the **ven**, get **thin**":

Stimulating **ven**tromedial increases satiety.

Lower vs. upper motor neuron lesion effects
1. "**STORM, Baby**"
2. 'In a **Lower** motor neuron lesion, everything goes **Down**:

STORM Baby tells you effects:

Strength

Tone

Other

Reflexes

Muscle mass

Babinski's sign

	Upper	Lower
Strength	▼	▼
Tone	▲ [spastic]	▼ [flaccid]
Other	fasiculations fibrillations clonus	
Reflexes	▲	▼
Muscle mass	slight loss only	▼
BABInski's sign	▲ [toe up]	▼ [toe down]

In Lower all things go down: strength, tone, reflexes, muscle mass, and the big toe down in plantar reflex (Babinski's sign is big toe up: toe up = UMNL).

See attached chart

Meninges: layers in order

PAD:

Piamater

Arachnoid

Dura

Olivary nuclei: ear vs. eye roles

Superior **O**livary nucleus: **SO**und localization.

Inferior olivary nucleus is therefore the one for sight [tactile, proprioception also].

Precentral vs. postcentral gyrus: motor vs. sensory

Just an extension of the rule that anterior = ventral = efferent = motor.

The precentral gyrus is on the anterior side of the brain, so is therefore motor.

Purkinje cells in cerebellum are inhibitory to deep nuclei

Shape of a purkinje cell in 3 dimensions is same as a policeman's hand saying "Stop".

Therefore, purkinje cells are inhibitory.

See diagram.

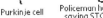

Purkinje cell   Policeman hand saying STOP!

Spinal cord: converting ventral/ anterior/ motor/ efferent and dorsal/ posterior/ sensory/ afferent

A limousine:

The **motor** of limo is **ventral** and **anterior** on the car.

The **A**erial is **sensory** and on the **dorsal** and **posterior** of the limo.

Note 1: '**A**' is **A**fferent, and also, in a limo, the aerial on the top of the trunk has a capital '**A**' shape.

Note 2: An aerial is a sensory thing: picks up radio waves.

Note 3: If picked a limo up in your hand, can only see motor on ventral, since dorsal is covered by thehood/bonnet.

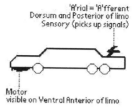

'A'rial = 'A'fferent
Dorsum and Posterior of limo
Sensory (picks up signals)

Motor
visible on Ventral Anterior of limo

Spinal tracts: Gracilus vs. Cuneatus: origin from upper vs. lower limbs

Gracilus is the name of a muscle in the legs, so Fasciculus **Gracilus** is for the lower limbs.

By default, Fasciculus Cuneatus must be for upper limbs.

Spinal tracts: simplified geography

2 posterior: cross at the medulla.
2 lateral: ipsilateral (same side).
2 anterior: cross at the spinal level.
  See diagram.

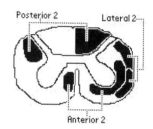

Posterior 2   Lateral 2

Anterior 2

Note 1: Descending tracts on left of figure, ascending tracts on right.
  Note 2: For ipsilaterals: one never crosses, one crosses at the level then doubles back farther up. The
  ipsilateral that crosses at the level (ventral spinocerebellar) is the ipsilateral closest to the 2 anterior ones,
  which also cross at the level.
  Tract names in each group:
Posterior 2: lateral corticalspinal, dorsal columns. Lateral 2: dorsal spinocerebellar, ventral spinocerebellar. Anterior 2: ventral corticospinal,spinothalamic.

Thirst/water balance control centre: location in hypothalamus

"You **look up** (supra...optic) at the clouds, to check if it's going to **rain** (water)":
Therefore, water balance is in supraoptic nucleus.

Ventricle aperatures: converting the two nomenclature types

Magendie foramen is the Medial aperture.
Luschka foramen is the Lateral aperture.

OBSTETRICS / GYNECOLOGY

Preeclampsia: classic triad

PREeclampsia:
Proteinuria
Rising blood pressure
Edema

RLQ pain: brief female differential

AEIOU:
Appendicitis/ Abscess
Ectopic pregnancy/ Endometriosis
Inflammatory disease (pelvic)/ IBD
Ovarian cyst (rupture, torsion)
Uteric colic/ Urinary stones

Abdominal pain: causes during pregnancy

LARA CROFT:
Labour
Abruption of placenta
Rupture (eg. ectopic/ uterus)
Abortion
Cholestasis

Rectus sheath haematoma
Ovarian tumour
Fibroids
Torsion of uterus

Alpha-fetoprotein: causes for increased maternal serum AFP during pregnancy

"Increased Maternal Serum Alpha Feto Protein":
Intestinal obstruction
Multiple gestation/ Miscalculation of gestational age/ Myeloschisis
Spina bifida cystica
Anencephaly/ Abdominal wall defect
Fetal death
Placental abruption

APGAR score components

SHIRT:
Skin color: blue or pink
Heart rate: below 100 or over 100
Irritability (response to stimulation): none, grimace or cry
Respirations: irregular or good
Tone (muscle): some flexion or active

Asherman syndrome features

ASHERMAN:
Acquired Anomaly
Secondary to Surgery
Hysterosalpingography confirms diagnosis
Endometrial damage/ Eugonadotropic
Repeated uterine trauma
Missed Menses
Adhesions
Normal estrogen and progesterone

B-agonist tocolytic (C/I or warning)

ABCDE:
Angina (Heart disease)
BP high
Chorioamnionitis
Diabetes
Excessive bleeding

CVS and amniocentesis: when performed

"Chorionic" has **9** letters and Chorionic villus sampling performed at **9** weeks gestation.
"AlphaFetoProtein" has **16** letters and it's measured at **16** weeks gestation.

Delivery: instrumental delivery prerequisites

AABBCCDDEE:
Analgesia
Antisepsis
Bowel empty
Bladder empty
Cephalic presentation
Consent
Dilated cervix
Disproportion (no CPD)
Engaged
Episiotomy

Dysfunctional uterine bleeding (DUB): 3 major causes

DUB:
Don't ovulate (anovulation: 90% of cases)
Unusual corpus leuteum activity (prolonged or insufficient)
Birth control pills (since increases progesterone-estrogen ratio)

Early cord clamping: indications

RAPID CS:

Rh incompatibility

Asphyxia

Premature delivery

Infections

Diabetic mother

CS (caesarian section) previously, so the funda is RAPID CS

Forceps: indications for delivery

FORCEPS:

Foetus alive

Os dilated

Ruptured membrane

Cervix taken up

Engagement of head

Presentation suitable

Sagittal suture in AP diameter of inlet

Forceps: indications for use

FORCEPS:

Fully dilated cervix

0 ["Zero"] CPD

Ruptured membranes

Cephalic or at least deliverable presentation/ Contracting uterus

Episiotomy done/ Epidural done

P!ss and S#!t (bladder and bowel empty)

IUD: side effects

PAINS:

Period that is late

Abdominal cramps

Increase in body temperature

Noticeable vaginal discharge

Spotting

IUGR: causes

IUGR:

Inherited: chromosomal and genetic disorders

Uterus: placental insufficency

General: maternal malnutrition, smoking

Rubella and other congenital infecton

Labour: preterm labor causes

DISEASE:

Dehydration

Infection

Sex

Exercise (strenuous)

Activities

Stress

Environmental factor (job, etc)

Multiple pregnancy complications

HI, PAPA:

Hydramnios (Poly)

IUGR

Preterm labour

Antepartum haemorrhage

Pre-eclampsia

Abortion

Omental caking: likeliest cause

Omental **CA**king = **O**varian **CA**

"Omental caking" is term for ascites, plus a fixed upper abdominal and pelvic mass. Almost always signifies ovarian cancer.

Oral contraceptive complications: warning signs
ACHES:

Abdominal pain

Chest pain

Headache (severe)

Eye (blurred vision)

Sharp leg pain

Oral contraceptives: side effects
CONTRACEPTIVES:

Cholestatic jaundice

Oedema (corneal)

Nasal congestion

Thyroid dysfunction

Raised BP

Acne/ Alopecia/ Anaemia

Cerebrovascular disease

Elevated blood sugar

Porphyria/ Pigmentation/ Pancreatitis

Thromboembolism

Intracranial hypertension

Vomiting (progesterone only)

Erythema nodosum/ Extrapyramidal effects

Sensitivity to light

Parity abbreviations (ie: G 3, P 2012)
"To Peace AndLove":

T: of Term pregnancies

P: of Premature births

A: of Abortions (spontaneous or elective)

L: of Live births

Describes the outcomes of the total number of pregnancies (Gravida).

Pelvic Inflammatory Disease (PID): causes, effects

"PID **CANbeEPIC**":

Causes:

Chlamydia trachomatis

Actinomycetes

Neisseria gonorrhoeae

Effects:

Ectopic

Pregnancy

Infertility

Chronic pain

Pelvic Inflammatory Disease (PID): complications

I FACE PID:

Infertility

Fitz-Hugh-Curitis syndrome

Abscesses

Chronic pelvic pain

Ectopic pregnancy

Peritonitis

Intestinal obstruction

Disseminated: sepsis, endocarditis, arthritis, meninigitis

Postpartum collapse: causes

HEPARINS:

Hemorrhage

Eclampsia

Pulmonary embolism

Amniotic fluid embolism

Regional anaethetic complications

Infarction (MI)

Neurogenic shock

Septic shock

Post-partum haemmorrage (PPH): risk factors
PARTUM:
Polyhydroamnios/ Prolonged labour/ Previous cesarian
APH/ ANTH
Recent bleeding history
Twins
Uterine fibroids
Multiparity

Prenatal care questions
ABCDE:
Amniotic fluid leakage?
Bleeding vaginally?
Contractions?
Dysuria?
Edema?
Fetal movement?

Secondary amenorrhea: causes
SOAP:
Stress
OCP
Anorexia
Pregnancy

Female pelvis: shapes
GAP:
In order from most to least common:
Gynecoid
Android /Anthropoid
Platypelloid

Red eye causes

GO SUCK:

Glaucoma
Orbital disease
Scleritis
Uveitis
Conjunctivitis
Keratitis

Cataracts: causes

ABCDE:

Aging
Bang: trauma, other injuries (eg infrared)
Congenital
Diabetes and other metabolic disturbances (eg steroids)
Eye diseases: glaucoma, uveitis

Cataracts: causes

CATARAct:

Congenital
Aging
Toxicity (steroids, etc)
Accidents
Radiation
Abnormal metabolism (diabetes mellitus, Wilson's)

Cataracts: differential

CATARAct:

Congenital
Aging
Toxicity (steroids, etc)

Accidents

Radiation

Abnormal metabolism (DM, Wilsons, etc)

Diplopia (uniocular): causes

ABCD:

Astigmatism

Behavioral: psychogenic

Cataract

Dislocated lens

Optic atrophy causes

ICING:

Ischaemia

Compressed nerve

Intracranial pressure [raised]

Neuritis history

Glaucoma

Periorbital cellulitis: etiology

SIGHT:

Sinusitis

Insect Bite

Globular/ Glandular Spread

Heme Spread

Trauma

Carpal tunnel syndrome: treatment
WRIST:
Wear splints at night
Rest
Inject steroid
Surgical decompression
Take diuretics

Fracture: how to describe
PLASTER OF PARIS:
Plane
Location
Articular cartilage involvement
Simple or comminuted
Type (eg Colles')
Extent
Reason
Open or closed
Foreign bodies
disPlacement
Angulation
Rotation
Impaction
Shortening

Bone fracture types [for Star Wars fans]
GO C3PO:
Greenstick
Open
Complete/ Closed/ Comminuted
Partial
Others
Note: C3P0 is droid in the Star-Wars movies.

Bryant's traction: position

BrYant's traction:

Bent Y.

Patient's body is the stem of the Y laying on the bed, and legs are the ends of the Y up in the air.

Monoarthritis differential

GHOST:

Gout

Haemarthrosis

Osteoarthritis

Sepsis

Trauma

Osteosarcoma: risk factors

PRIMARY:

Paget's

Radiation

Infaction of bone

Male

Alcohol, poor diet, sedentary lifestyle [adults only]

Retinoblastoma, Li-Fraumeni syndrome

Young [10-20 yrs]

Osteosarcoma is the most common **primary** malignant tumor of bone.

Pagets disease of bone: signs and symptoms

PANICS:

Pain

Arthralgia

Nerve compression / Neural deafness

Increased bone density

Cardiac failure

Skull / Sclerotic vertebrae

Achalasia: 1 possible cause, 1 treatment

a**CHA**lasia:

1 possible cause: **CHA**gas' disease

1 treatment: Ca++ **CHA**nnel blockers

Carcinoid syndrome: components

CARCinoid:

Cutaneous flushing

Asthmatic wheezing

Right sided valvular heart lesions

Cramping and diarrhea

Gallstones: risk factors

5 F's:

Fat

Female

Family history

Fertile

Forty

Haemochromatosis definition, classic triad

"**Iron man tri**athalon":

Iron man: deposition of **iron** in many body tissues.

Triathalon has 3 components, which match **tri**ad:

Swimming: **S**kin pigmentation

Biking: **B**ronze diabetes

Marathon: **M**icronodular pigment cirrhosis

See diagram for visual equivalent.

Triathlete:

Black athlete:
skin pigmentation

Bronze medal:
bronze diabetes

Liver dots:
micronodular
pigment cirrhosis

Hepatomegaly: 3 common causes, 3 rarer causes

Common are 3 C's:

Cirrhosis

Carcinoma

Cardiac failure

Rarer are 3 C's:

Cholestasis

Cysts

Cellular infiltration

IBD: extraintestinal manifestations

"Left intestine to sail the **SEAS** of the rest of the body":

Skin manifestations: erythema nodosum, pyoderma gangrenosum

Eye inflammation: iritis, episcleritis

Arthritis

Sclerosing cholangitis

Inflammatory Bowel Disease: which has cobblestones

Crohn's has Cobblestones on endoscopy.

Kwashiorkor: distinguishing from Marasmus

FLAME:

Fatty Liver

Anemia

Malabsorption

Edema

Pancreatitis: causes

PANCREATITIS:

Posterior

Alcohol

Neoplasm

Cholelithiasis

Rx (lasix, AZT)
ERCP
Abdominal surgery
Trauma
Infection (mumps)
Triglycerides elevated
Idiopathic
Scorpion bite

PKU findings

PKU:
Pale hair, skin
Krazy (neurological abnormalities)
Unpleasant smell

Ulcerative colitis: features

ULCERATIONS:
Ulcers
Large intestine
Carcinoma [risk]
Extraintestinal manifestations
Remnants of old ulcers [pseudopolyps]
Abscesses in crypts
Toxic megacolon [risk]
Inflamed, red, granular mucosa
Originates at rectum
Neutrophil invasion
Stools bloody

Acute ischemia: signs [especially limbs]

6 P's:

Pain

Pallor

Pulselessness

Paralysis

Paraesthesia

Perishingly cold

Anemia (normocytic): causes

ABCD:

Acute blood loss

Bone marrow failure

Chronic disease

Destruction (hemolysis)

Anemia causes (simplified)

ANEMIA:

Anemia of chronic disease

No folate or B12

Ethanol

Marrow failure & hemaglobinopathies

Iron deficient

Acute & chronic blood loss

Aneurysm types

MAD SCAB:

Mycotic

Atherosclerotic

Dissecting

Syphilitic

Capillary microaneurysm

Arteriovenous fistula

Berry

Atherosclerosis risk factors

"You're a **SAD BET** with these risk factors":

Sex: male

Age: middle-aged, elderly

Diabetes mellitus

BP high: hypertension

Elevated cholesterol

Tobacco

Blood disorders: commoner sex

HE (male) gets:

HEmophilia (X-linked)

HEinz bodies (G6PD deficiency, causing **HE**molytic anemia: X-linked)

HEmochromatosis (male predominance)

HEart attacks (male predominance)

HEnoch-Schonlein purpura (male predominance)

SHE (female) gets:

SHEehan's syndrome

Buerger's disease features

"**burger SCRAPS**":

Segmenting thrombosing vasculitis

Claudication (intermittent)

Raynaud's phenomenon

Associated with smoking

Pain, even at rest

Superficial nodular phlebitis

Alternatively, if hungry for more detail [sic], "**CRISP PIG burgers**":

Chronic ulceration

Raynaud's phenomenon

Intermittent claudication
Segmenting, thrombosing vasculitis
Pain, even at rest
Phlebitis (superficial nodular)
Idiopathic
Gangrene

Cardiovascular risk factors

FLASH BODIES:

Family history
Lipids
Age
Sex
Homocystinaemia
Blood pressure
Obesity
Diabetes mellitus
Inflammation (raised CRP)/ increased thrombosis
Exercise
Smoking

Deep venous thrombosis: diagnosis

DVT:

Dilated superficial veins/ Discoloration/ Doppler ultrasound
Venography is gold standard
Tenderness of Thigh and calf

Disseminated Intravascular Cogulation: causes

DIC:

Delivery **TEAR** (obstetric complications)
Infections (gram negative)/ Immunological
Cancer (prostate, pancreas, lung, stomach)
Obstretrical complications are **TEAR**:

Toxemia of pregnancy
Emboli (amniotic)
Abrutio placentae
Retain fetus products

Fat embolism: findings

"**Fat**, **Bat**, **Fract**":
Fat in urine, sputum
Bat-wing lung x-ray
Fracture history
    Also, fracture of **FEM**ur causes **Fat EMb**oli.

Heart failure causes

"**HEART MAy DIE**":
Hypertension
Embolism
Anemia
Rheumatic heart disease
Thyrotoxicosis (incl. pregnancy)
Myocardial infarct
Arrythmia
Y
Diet & lifestyle
Infection
Endocarditis

Hypertension: secondary hypertension causes

CHAPS:
Cushing's syndrome
Hyperaldosteronism [aka Conn's syndrome]
Aorta coarctation
Phaeochromocytoma
Stenosis of renal arteries

Note: only 5% of hypertension cases are secondary, rest are primary.

Kawasaki disease: diagnostic criteria
CHILD:

5 letters=**5** days, >**5** years old, **5** out 6 criteria for diagnosis:
Conjuctivitis (bilateral)
Hyperthermia (fever) >5 days
Idiopathic polymorphic rash
Lymphoadenopathy (cervical)
Dryness & redness of (i)lips& month (ii)palms & soles [2 separate criteria]

Kawasaki disease: features
Disease name: a Kawasaki motorcycle.
Usually young children, epidemic in Japan: Japanese child rides the motorcycle.
Conjunctival, oral erythema: red eyes, mouth.
Fever: thermometer.
Erythema of palms, soles: red palms, soles.
Generalized rash: rash dots.
Cervical lymphadenitis: enlarged cervical nodes with inflammation arrows.
Vasculitis of arteries: inflammation arrows on arteries.
Cardiovascular sequelae [20%]: inflammation arrows on cardiac arteries.
Treat with aspirin: aspirin headlight.
See diagram.

MI: complications
HAS CRAPPED:
Heart failure/ **H**ypertension
Arrhythmia
Shock
Cardiac **R**upture
Aneurysm
Pericarditis
Pulmonary Emboli
DVT

MI: post-MI complications
ACT RAPID:
Arrhythmias (SVT, VT, VF)
Congestive cardiac failure
Tamponade/ **T**hromboembolic disorders
Rupture (ventricle, septum, papillary muscle)
Aneurysm (ventricle)
Pericarditis
Infaction (a second one)
Death/ **D**ressler's syndrome

MI: sequence of elevated enzymes after MI
"Time to **CAL**L 911":
   From first to appear to last:
Troponin
CK-MB
AST
LDH1

Pericarditis: findings

PERICarditis:

Pulsus paradoxus

ECG changes

Rub

Increased JVP

Chest pain [worse on inspiration, better when lean forward]

Pick's disease: location, action, epidemiology

Pick axes are **Pick**ing away at the old woman's cerebral cortex, causing cortical atrophy.

2 pick axes on her brain: frontal lobe and anterior 1/3 of temporal. An old woman, since epidemiology is elderly & more common in women. See figure.

Takayasu's disease is Pulseless disease

"Can't **Tak'a yapulse**" (Can't take your pulse):

Takayasu's disease known as Pulseless disease, since pulse is weakened in the upper extremities.

Thrombotic thrombocytopenic purpura: signs

FAT RN:

Fever

Anemia

Thrombocytopenia

Renal problems

Neurologic dysfunction

TTP: clinical features

Thrombosis and thrombocytopenia **PARTNER** together:
Platelet count low
Anemia (microangiopathic hemolytic)
Renal failure
Temperature rise
Neurological deficits
ER admission (as it is an emergency)

Virchow's triad (venous thrombosis)

"**VIR**chow":
Vascular trauma
Increased coagulability
Reduced blood flow (stasis)

Von Hippel-Lindau: signs and symptoms

HIPPEL:
Hemanigoblastomas
Increased renal cancer
Pheochromocytoma
Port-wine stains
Eye dysfunction
Liver, pancreas, kidney cysts
    Bare bones version: Hippel-Lindau, with H and L as above.

Addison's disease: features

ADDISON:
Autoimmune
DIC (meningcoccus)
Destruction by cancer, infection, vascular insufficiency
Iatrogenic
Sarcoidosis, granulomatous such as TB histiomycosis
hyp**O**tension/ hyp**O**natermia
Nelson's syndrome [post adrelectomy, increased ACTH]

Cushing syndrome
CUSHING:

Central obesity/ Cervical fat pads/ Collagen fiber weakness/ Comedones (acne)

Urinary free corisol and glucose increase

Striae/ Suppressed immunity

Hypercortisolism/ Hypertension/ Hyperglycemia/ Hirsutism

Iatrogenic (Increased administration of corticosteroids)

Noniatrogenic (Neoplasms)

Glucose intolerance/ Growth retardation

Goitre: differential
GOITRE:

Goitrogens

Onset of puberty

Iodine deficiency

Thyrotoxicosis/ Tumor/ Thyroiditis [Hashimoto's]

Reproduction [pregnancy]

Enzyme deficiencies

Hirsutism vs. virilism

Hirsutism: Hair on body like a male.

Virilism: Voice and rest of secondary sexual characteristics like a male.

Hypercalcemia: symptoms of elevated serum levels
"Bones, Stones, Groans, Moans":

Bones: pain in bones

Stones: renal

Groans: pain

Psychic **moans**/ Psychological **overtones**: confused state

Multiple endocrine neoplasia III: components

MEN III is a disease of **3 M's**:

Medullary thyroid carcinoma

Medulla of adrenal (pheochromocytoma)

Mucosal neuroma

Pheochromocytoma: 3 most common symptoms

"**PHE**ochromocytoma":

Palpitations

Headache

Edisodic sweating (diaphoresis)

Thyroid carcinoma: features, prognosis of most popular

Most **P**opular is **P**apillary.

Clinical features:

Papillae (branching)

Palpable lymph nodes

"**P**upil" nuclei (Orphan Annie)

Psammoma bodies within lesion (often)

Also, has a **P**ositive **P**rognosis (10 year survival rate: 98%).

Thyroid storm characteristics

"**Storm HITS girls cAMP**":

Thyroid **storm** due to:

Hyperthyroidism

Infection or **I**llness at childbirth

Trauma

Surgery

girls: Thyroid storm more common in females.

cAMP: Tx involves high dose of beta blockers (beta receptors work via cAMP)

Alternatively: "**S#IT storm**": Surgery, Hyperthyroidism, Infection/ Illness, Trauma.

Baldness risk factors

"**D**addy **D**oesn't **D**eny **G**etting **H**air **I**mplants":

Diet

Disease

Drugs

Genes

Hormones

Injury to the scalp

Diabetic ketoacidosis: I vs. II

ket**ONE** bodies are seen in type **ONE** diabetes.

Lichen planus characteristics

Planus has 4 **P**'s:

Peripheral

Polygonal

Pruritus

Purple

APKD: signs, complications, accelerators

11 **B**'s:

  Signs:

Bloody urine

Bilateral pain [vs. stones, which are usually unilateral pain]

Blood pressure up

Bigger kidneys

Bumps palpable

  Complications:

Berry aneurysm

Biliary cysts

Bicuspid valve [prolapse and other problems]

  Accelerators:

Boys

Blacks

Blood pressure high

Gout vs. pseudogout: crystal lab findings

Pseduogout crystals are:

Positive birefringent

Polygon shaped

Gout therefore is the negative needle shaped crystals.

Also, gout classically strikes great **Toe**, and its hallmark is **To**phi.

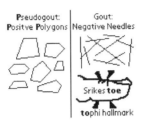

Gout: factors that can precipitate an attack of acute gouty arthritis

DARK:

Diuretics

Alcohol

Renal disease

Kicked (trauma)

And, the attack occurs most often at night [thus "dark"].

Gout: major features

GOUT:

Great toe

One joint (75% monoarticular)

Uric acid increased (hence urolithiasis)

Tophi

Hematuria: urethral causes

NUTS:

Neoplasm

Urethritis
Tumour
Stone

Nephritic syndrome: glomerular diseases commonly presenting as nephritic syndrome
PARIS:
Post-streptococcal
Alport's
RPGN
IgA nephropathy
SLE
Alternatively: **PIG ARMS** to include Goodpasture's [one cause of RPGN], Membranoproliferative [only sometimes included in the classic nephritic list].

Nephrotic syndrome: hallmark findings
"**Protein LEAC**":
Proteinuria
Lipid up
Edema
Albumin down
Cholesterol up
In nephrotic, the **proteins leak** out.

Renal failure (chronic): consequences
ABCDEFG:
Anemia
-due to less EPO
Bone alterations
-osteomalacia
-osteoporosis
-von Recklinghausen
Cardiopulmonary

-atherosclerosis
-CHF
-hypertension
-pericarditis
D vitamin loss
Electrolyte imbalance
-sodium loss/gain
-metabolic acidosis
-hyperkalemia
Feverous infections
-due to leukocyte abnormalities and dialysis hazards
GI disturbances
-haemorrhagic gastritis
-peptic ulcer disease
-intractable hiccups

Renal failure: causes
AVID GUT:
Acute tubular necrosis
Vascular obstruction
Infection
Diffuse intravascular coagulation
Glomerular disease
Urinary obstruction
Tubulointerstitial nephritis

Anemia: TIBC finding to differentiate iron deficiency vs. chronic disease
TIBC levels at the:
Top=Iron deficiency.
Bottom=Chronic disease.

Hemophilia: type A factor

Hemophilia **A**: problems with VIII factor (number **V** as an inverted **A**).

Leukemias: acute vs. chronic rules of thumb

ABCDE:

Acute is:

Blasts predominate

Children

Drastic course

Elderly

Few WBC's (so **F**evers)

   Chronic is all the opposites:

Mature cells predominate

Middle aged

Less debilitating course

Elevated WBC's, so not a history of fevers and infections

Megaloblastic anemia: vitamin B12 deficiency vs. folate deficiency

Vitamin **B**12 deficiency also affects **B**rain (optic neuropathy, subacute combined degeneration, paresthesia).

   Folate deficiency is not associated with neurological symptoms.

Sarcoidosis summarized

SARCOIDOISIS:

Schaumann calcifications

Asteroid bodies/ [ACE] increase/ **A**nergy

Respiratory complications/ **R**enal calculi/ **R**estrictive lung disease/ **R**estrictive cardiomyopathy

Calcium increase in serum and urine/ **C**D4 helper cells

Ocular lesions

Immune mediated noncaseating granulomas/ [**I**g] increase

Diabetes insipidus/ [**D** vit.] increase/ **D**yspnea

Osteopathy

Skin (Subcutaneous nodules, erythema nodosum)
Interstitial lung fibrosis/ IL-1
Seventh CN palsy

Wiskott-Aldrich syndrome: symptom triad
"**PET** WASP":
Pyrogenic infections
Eczema
Thrombocytopenia
   WASP is the name of the causitive agent: Wiskott-Aldrich
   Syndrome Protein.
   Alternatively: Wiskott=Hot, Aldrich=Itch, Syndrom=Throm.

Duchenne vs. Becker Muscular Dystrophy
Duchenne **M**uscular **D**ystrophy (DMD) :**D**oesn't **M**ake **D**ystrophin.
Becker **M**uscular **D**ystrophy (BMD): **B**adly **M**ade **D**ystrophin (a
truncated protein).

McArdle's syndrome
MCARDLES:
Myoglobinuria
Cramping after exercise
Accumulated glycogen
Recessive inheritance
Deficiency of muscle phosphorylase
Lactate levels fail to rise
Elevated creatine kinase
Skeletal muscle only

Alzheimer's disease (AD): associations, findings

AD:
   Associations:
Aluminum toxicity
Acetylcholine deficiencies
Amyloid B
Apolipoprotein gene E
Altered nucleus basalis of Meynert
Down's
   Findings:
Actin inclusions (Hirano bodies)
Atrophy of brain
Amyloid plaques
Aphasia, **A**praxia, **A**gitation
DNA-coiled tangles
Dementia, **D**isoriented, **D**epressed

Cerebral palsy: general features

PALSY:
Paresis
Ataxia
Lagging motor development
Spasticity
Young

Lou Gehrig's is both upper and lower motor neuron signs

Lo**U** = **L**ower & **U**pper.

Parkinsonism: essential features

TRAPS:
Tremor (resting tremor)
Rigidity

Akinesia

Postural changes (stooped)

Stare (serpentine stare)

To remember what kind of tremor and postural change, can look at letter that follows in TRAPS: Tremor is Resting, Posture is Stooped.

Pyrogenic meningitis: likeliest bug in age group

"Explaining Hot Neck Stiffness":

In order from birth to death:

E. coli [infants]

Haemophilus influenzae [older infants, kids]

Neisseria meningitis [young adults]

Streptococcus pneumoniae [old folks]

Tabes Dorsalis morphology

DORSALIS:

Dorsal column degeneration

Orthopedic pain (Charcot joints)

Reflexes decreased (deep tendon)

Shooting pain

Argyll-Robertson pupils

Locomotor ataxia

Impaired proprioception

Syphilis

Tuberous sclerosis: presenting features

"Zits, Fits, Deficits":

Fits: seizures

Deficits: neurological deficits

Wernicke-Korsakoff's psychosis: findings

COAT RACK:

Wernicke's encephalopathy (acute phase):

Confusion

Ophthalmoplegia

Ataxia

Thiamine tx.

Korsakoff's psychosis (chronic phase):

Retrograde amnesia

Anterograde amnesia

Confabulation

Korsakoff's psychosis

Edwards' syndrome: characteristics

EDWARDS:

Eighteen (trisomy)

Digit overlapping flexion

Wide head

Absent intellect (mentally retarded)

Rocker-bottom feet

Diseased heart

Small lower jaw

Fragile X syndrome: features

FEMALES

FMR1 gene

Exhibits anticpation

Macro-orchidism

Autism

Long face with large jaw

Everted eyes

Second most common casue of genetic mental retardation

Fragile-X syndrome: features

DSM-4:

Discontinued chromosome staining

Shows anticipation

Male (male more affected)

Mental retardation (2nd most common genetic cause)

Macrognathia

Macroorchidism

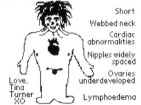

Turner syndrome: components

CLOWNS:

Cardiac abnormalities (specifically **C**oartication)

Lymphoedema

Ovaries underdeveloped (causing sterility, amenorrhea)

Webbed neck

Nipples widely spaced

Short

Bronchial obstruction: consequences

APPLE BABE:

Atelectasis

Pleural adhesions

Pleuritis

Lipid pneumonia

Effusion->organisation->fibrosis

Bronchiectasis

Abscess

Broncho and lobar pneumonia

Emphysema

COPD: 4 types and hallmark

ABCDE:

Asthma

Brochiectasis

Chronic bronchitis
Dyspnea [hallmark of group]
Emphysema
Alternatively: replace Dyspnea with Decreased FEV1/FVC ratio.

COPD: blue bloater vs. pink puffer diseases
emPhysema has letter P (and not B) so Pink Puffer.
chronicBronchitis has letter B (and not P) so Blue Bloater.

Emphysema: types, most important feature of each
"Cigarettes Is Primary Problem":
Types:
Centrilobular
Irregular
Pancinar
Paraseptal
Most important feature for each type (in order as above):
Cigarrettes
Inflammation healed to scar
Protease inhibitor deficiency (a1-antitrypsin)
Pneumothorax
"Cigarettes is primary problem" used since cigarettes is most common cause of emphysema.
Keeping P's straight: Pan is antitrypsin.

Interstitial lung disease: causes
SARCOIDI:
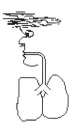
Sarcoidosis
Allergic reaction
Radiation
Connective tissue disease
Occupational exposure
Infection

Drugs
Idiopathic

Nasopharyngeal malignant cancers

NASOPharyngeal:
Nasophayngeal
Adenocarcinoma
Squamous cell carcinoma
Olfactory neuroblastoma
Plasmacytoma

Pancoast tumor: relationship with Horner's syndrome

"**Horner** has a **MAP** of the **Coast**":
A pan**Coast** tumor is a cancer of the lung apex that compresses the cervical sympathetic plexus, causing **Horner**'s syndrome, which is MAP:
Miosis
Anhidrosis
Ptosis

Pneumothorax: presentation

P-THORAX:
Pleuretic pain
Trachea deviation
Hyperresonance
Onset sudden
Reduced breath sounds (& dypsnea)
Absent fremitus
X-ray shows collapse
Dublin

Pulmonary embolism: risk factors
TOM SCHREPFER:
Trauma
Obesity
Malignancy
Surgery
Cardiac disease
Hospitalization
Rest [bed-ridden]
Elderly
Past history
Fracture
Estrogen [pregnancy, post-partum]
Road trip

Respiratory distress syndrome in infants: major risk factors
PCD (Primary Ciliary Dyskinesia, a cause of Respiratory distress syndrome):
Prematurity
Cesarean section
Diabetic mother

TB: features
TB is characterised by 4 C's:
Caseation
Calcification
Cavitation
Cicatrization

Breast cancer: risk assessment
"Risk can be assessed by **History ALONE**":
History (family, previous episode)
Abortion/ **Age** (old)

Late menopause
Obesity
Nulliparity
Early menarche

Endometrial carcinoma: risk factors

ENDOMET:

Elderly
Nulliparity
Diabetes
Obesity
Menstrual irregularity
Estrogen therapy
hyperTension

Polycystic ovary: morphology, presentation

TB: features

TB is characterised by 4 C's:

Caseation
Calcification
Cavitation
Cicatrization
Knowledge Level 3, System: Pulmonary
Sameh Shehata Asst. Prof of Surgery, Faculty of Medicine,
University of Alexandria, Egypt
   Morphology is **poly-C**:
Cysts
Capsule thickened
Cortical stromal fibrosis
   Clinical presentation is **OVARY**:
Obese
Virilism or hirsutism
Amenorrhoea

Reproductive problem [infertile]
Young woman

Scrotum masses
SHOVE IT:
Spermatocele
Hydrocele/ Haematocele
Orchitis
Varicocele
Epidymal cyst
Indirect inguinal hernia
Torsion/ Tumor

Carcinomas having tendency to metastasize to bone
"Kinds OfTumors Leaping Primarily To Bone":
Kidneys
Ovaries
Testes
Lungs
Prostate
Thyroid
Breasts
Alternatively: "Promptly" instead of "Primarily".
Alternatively: "BLT2 with a Kosher Pickle".

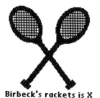

Histiocytosis X: hallmark finding
Birbeck's rackets is X

"Birbeck's rackets is X":
Tennis rackets under electron microscope is Histiocystosis X.
Consider 2 tennis rackets in an X formation.
See diagram.

Marble bone disease: signs and symptoms

MARBLES:

Multiple fractures

Anemia

Restricted cranial nerves

Blind & deaf

Liver enlarged

Erlenmeyer flask deformity

Splenomegaly

Eponymous name: **Marbles** = **Albers**-Schonberg (anagram).

Paget's disease of bone: signs and symptoms

Four L's:

Larger hat size

Loss of hearing: due to compression of nerve

Leontiasis ossea (lion-like face)

Light-headed (Paget's steal)

PEDIATRICS

Duodenal atresia vs. Pyloric stenosis: site of obstruction

Duodenal Atresia: **D**istal to Ampulla of vater.

Pyloric stenosis: Proximal to it.

Pyloric stenosis (congential): presentation

Pyloric stenosis is 3 **P**'s:

Palpable mass

Paristalsis visible

Projectile vomiting (2-4 weeks after birth)

Vitamin toxicities: neonatal
Excess vitamin **A**: **A**nomalies (teratogenic)
Excess vitamin **E**: **E**nterocolitis (necrotizing enterocolitis)
Excess vitamin **K**: **K**ernicterus (hemolysis)

Cyanotic congenital heart diseases
5 T's:
Truncus arteriosus
Transposition of the great arteries
Tricuspid atresia
Tetrology of Fallot
Total anomalous pulmonary venous return

Cyanotic heart diseases: 5 types
Use your five fingers:
1 finger up: Truncus Arteriosus (**1** vessel)
2 fingers up: Dextroposition of the Great Arteries (**2** vessels transposed)
3 fingers up: Tricuspid Atresia (**3**=Tri)
4 fingers up: Tetralogy of Fallot (**4**=Tetra)
5 fingers up: Total Anomalous Pulmonary Venous Return (**5**=5 words)

Hemolytic-Uremic Syndrome (HUS): components
"Remember to decrease the **RATE** of IV fluids in these patients":
Renal failure
Anemia (microangiopathic, hemolytic)
Thrombocytopenia
Encephalopathy (TTP)

Haematuria: differential in children

ABCDEFGHIJK:

Anatomy (cysts, etc)

Bladder (cystitis)

Cancer (Wilm's tumour)

Drug related (cyclophosphamide)

Exercise induced

Factitious (Munchausen by proxy)

Glomerulonephritis

Haematology (bleeding disorder, sickle cell)

Infection (UTI)

In Jury (trauma)

Kidney stones (hypercalciuria)

Perez reflex

Eliciting the **PErEz** reflex will make the baby **PEE**.

Cerebral palsy (CP): most likely cause

CP: **C**erebral **P**alsy

Child **P**remature

The premature brain is more prone to all the possible insults.

Pediatric milestones in development

1 year:

-**single** words

2 years:

-**2** word sentences

-understands **2** step commands

3 years:

-**3** word combos

-repeats **3** digits

-rides **tri**cycle

4 years:

-draws **square**

-counts **4** objects

Sturge-Weber syndrome: hallmark features
Sturge-Weber:
1. Seizures
2. PortWine stain

Guthrie card: diseases identified with it
"**G**uthrie **C**ards **C**an **H**elp **P**redict **B**ad **M**etabolism":
Galactosaemia
Cystic fibrosis
Congenital adrenal hyperplasia
Hypothyroidism
Phenylketonuria
Biotidinase deficiency
Maple syrup urine disease

Measles: complications
"**MEASLES COMP**" (complications):
Myocarditis
Encephalitis
Appendicitis
Subacute sclerosing panencephalitis
Laryngitis
Early death
Sh!ts (diarrhoea)
Corneal ulcer
Otis media
Mesenteric lymphadenitis
Pneumonia and related (bronchiolitis-bronchitis-croup)

Russell Silver syndrome: features

ABCDEF:

Asymmetric limb (hemihypertrophy)

Bossing (frontal)

Clinodactyly/ **C**afe au lait spots

Dwarf (short stature)

Excretion (GU malformation)

Face (triangular face, micrognathia)

Williams syndrome: features

WILLIAMS:

Weight (low at birth, slow to gain)

Iris (stellate iris)

Long philtrum

Large mouth

Increased Ca++

Aortic stenosis (and other stenoses)

Mental retardation

Swelling around eyes (periorbital puffiness)

Cough (chronic): differential

When cough in nursery, rock the **"CRADLE"**:

Cystic fibrosis

Rings, slings, and airway things (tracheal rings)/ **R**espiratory infections

Aspiration (swallowing dysfunction, TE fistula, gastroesphageal reflux)

Dyskinetic cilia

Lung, airway, and vascular malformations (tracheomalacia, vocal cord dysfunction)

Edema (heart failure)

Croup: symptoms

3 S's:
Stridor
Subglottic swelling
Seal-bark cough

Cystic fibrosis: exacerbation of pulmonary infection

CF PANCREAS:

Cough (increase in intensity and frequent spells)
Fever (usually low grade, unless severe bronchopneumonia is present)
Pulmonary function deterioration
Appetite decrease
Nutrition, weight loss
CBC (leukocytosis with left shift)
Radiograph (increase overaeration, peribronchial thickening, mucus plugging)
Exam (rales or wheezing in previously clear areas, tachypnea, retractions)
Activity (decreased, impaired exercise intolerance, increased absenteeism)
Sputum (becomes darker, thicker, and more abundant, forming plugs)

Cystic fibrosis: presenting signs

CF PANCREAS:

Chronic cough and wheezing
Failure to thrive
Pancreatic insufficiency (symptoms of malabsorption like steatorrhea)
Alkalosis and hypotonic dehydration
Neonatal intestinal obstruction (meconium ileus)/ Nasal polyps
Clubbing of fingers/ Chest radiograph with characteristic changes

Rectal prolapse
Electrolyte elevation in sweat, salty skin
Absence or congenital atresia of vas deferens
Sputum with Staph or Pseudomonas (mucoid)

Breast feeding: benefits
ABCDEFGH:
  Infant:
Allergic condition reduced
Best food for infant
Close relationship with mother
Development of IQ, jaws, mouth
  Mother:
Econmical
Fitness: quick return to pre-pregnancy body shape
Guards against cancer: breast, ovary, uterus
Hemorrhage (postpartum) reduced

Septic Arthritis: most common cause
Staphylococcus **A**ureus is the most common cause of
Septic **A**rthritis in the pediatric population.

PHARMACOLOGY

Hepatic necrosis: drugs causing focal to massive necrosis
"Very Angry Hepatocytes":
Valproic acid
Acetaminophen
Halothane

Adrenoceptors: vasomotor function of alpha vs. beta

ABCD:

Alpha = **C**onstrict.

Beta = **D**ilate.

Antiarrhythmics: class III members

BIAS:

Bretylium

Ibutilide

Amiodarone

Sotalol

Beta blockers with intrinsic sympathomimetic activity

Picture **diabetic** and **asthmatic** kids riding away on a **cart** that rolls on **pin**wheels.

Pindolol and **Cart**eolol have high and moderate ISA respectively, making them acceptable for use in some

diabetics or asthmatics despite the fact that they are non-selective beta blockers.

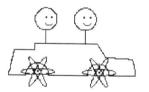

Beta-blockers: main contraindications, cautions

ABCDE:

Asthma

Block (heart block)

COPD

Diabetes mellitus

Electrolyte (hyperkalemia)

Beta-blockers: nonselective beta-blockers

"**TimPin**ches **HisNa**sal **Pro**blem" (because he has a runny nose...):

Timolol

Pindolol

Hismolol

Naldolol

Propranolol

Captopril (an ACE inhibitor): side effects

CAPTOPRIL:

Cough

Angioedema/ **A**granulocystosis

Proteinuria/ **P**otassium excess

Taste changes

Orthostatic hypotension

Pregnancy contraindication/ **P**ancreatitis/ **P**ressure drop (first dose hypertension)

Renal failure (and renal artery stenosis contraindication)/ **R**ash

Indomethacin inhibition

Leukopenia/ **L**iver toxicity

Enoxaprin (prototype low molecular weight heparin): action, monitoring

Eno**X**aprin only acts on factor **Xa**.

Monitor **Xa** concentration, rather than APTT.

HMG-CoA reductase inhibitors (statins): side effects, contraindications, interactions

HMG-CoA:

  Side effects:

Hepatotoxicity

Myositis [aka rhabdomyolysis]

  Contraindications:

Girl during pregnancy/ **G**rowing children

  Interactions:

Coumarin/ Cyclosporine

Hypertension: treatment
ABCD:
ACE inhibitors/ **A**ngII antagonists (sometimes **A**lpha agonists also)
Beta blockers
Calcium antagonists
Diuretics

Patent ductus arteriosus: treatment
"Come **In** and **Close** the door":
INdomethacin is used to **Close** PDA.

Propranolol and related '-olol' drugs: usage
"**olol**" is just two backwards lower case b's.
Backward b's stand for "**beta blocker**".
Beta blockers include acebut**olol**, betax**olol**, bisop**rolol**, oxpren**olol**, propran**olol**.

Thrombolytic agents
USA:
Urokinase
Streptokinase
Alteplase (tPA)

Warfarin: action, monitoring
WePT:
Warfarin works on the **e**xtrinsic pathway and is monitored by **PT**.

Warfarin: metabolism
SLOW:
Has a **slow** onset of action.
A quic**K** Vitamin **K** antagonist, though.

Small lipid-soluble molecule
Liver: site of action
Oral route of administration.
Warfarin

Gynaecomastia-causing drugs
DISCOS:
Digoxin
Isoniazid
Spironolactone
Cimetidine
Oestrogens
Stilboestrol

K+ increasing agents
K-BANK:
K-sparing diuretic
Beta blocker
ACEI
NSAID
K supplement

Propythiouracil (PTU): mechanism
It inhibits **PTU**:
Peroxidase/ **P**eripheral deiodination
Tyrosine iodination
Union (coupling)

Steroid side effects
CUSHINGOID:
Cataracts
Ulcers
Skin: striae, thinning, bruising

Hypertension/ Hirsutism/ Hyperglycemia
Infections
Necrosis, avascular necrosis of the femoral head
Glycosuria
Osteoporosis, obesity
Immunosuppression
Diabetes

Steroids: side effects
BECLOMETHASONE:
Buffalo hump
Easy bruising
Cataracts
Larger appetite
Obesity
Moonface
Euphoria
Thin arms & legs
Hypertension/ Hyperglycaemia
Avascular necrosis of femoral head
Skin thinning
Osteoporosis
Negative nitrogen balance
Emotional liability

Lupus: drugs inducing it
HIP:
Hydralazine
INH
Procanimide

Diuretics: thiazides: indications

"**CHIC** to use thiazides":
CHF
Hypertension
Insipidous
Calcium calculi

Nitrofurantoin: major side effects

Nitro**F**ur**A**ntoin:
Neuropathy (peripheral neuropathy)
Fibrosis (pulmonary fibrosis)
Anemia (hemolytic anemia)

Osmotic diuretics: members

GUM:
Glycerol
Urea
Mannitol

SIADH-inducing drugs

ABCD:
Analgesics: opioids, NSAIDs
Barbiturates
Cyclophosphamide/ **C**hlorpromazine/ **C**arbamazepine
Diuretic (thiazide)

Sulfonamide: major side effects

Sulfonamide side effects:
Steven-Johnson syndrome
Skin rash
Solubility low (causes crystalluria)
Serum albumin displaced (causes newborn kernicterus and potentiation of other serum albumin-binders like warfarin)

Vir-named drugs: use

"**-vir** at start, middle or end means for **virus**":
Drugs: Abaca**vir**, Acyclo**vir**, Amprena**vir**, Cidofo**vir**, Dena**vir**, Efa**vir**enz, Inda**vir**, In**vir**ase, Fam**vir**, Ganciclo**vir**, Nor**vir**, Oseltami**vir**, Penciclo**vir**, Ritona**vir**, Saquina**vir**, Valacyclo**vir**, **Vir**acept, **Vir**amune, Zanami**vir**, Zo**vir**ax.

4-Aminopyradine (4-AP) use

"**4-AP** is **For AP**":
For AP (action potential) propagation in Multiple Sclerosis.

Anticholinergic side effects

"Know the **ABCD'S** of anticholinergic side effects":
Anorexia
Blurry vision
Constipation/ **C**onfusion
Dry Mouth
Sedation/ **S**tasis of urine

Antimuscarinics: members, action

"**I**nhibits **P**arasympathetic **A**nd **S**weat":
Ipratropium
Pirenzepine
Atropine
Scopolamine
Muscarinic receptors at all parasympathetic endings sweat glands in sympathetic.

Aspirin: side effects

ASPIRIN:
Asthma
Salicyalism

Peptic ulcer disease/ Phosphorylation-oxidation uncoupling/ PPH/
Platelet disaggregation/ Premature closure of PDA
Intestinal blood loss
Reye's syndrome
Idiosyncracy
Noise (tinnitus)

Benzodiazapines: ones not metabolized by the liver (safe to use in liver failure)

LOT:
Lorazepam
Oxazepam
Temazepam

Benzodiazepenes: antidote

"**Ben** is **off** with the **flu**":
Benzodiazepine effects **off** with **Flu**mazenil.

Benzodiazepenes: drugs which decrease their metabolism

"**I**'m **O**verly **C**alm":
Isoniazid
Oral contraceptive pills
Cimetidine
These drugs increase calming effect of BZDs by retarding metabolism.

Benzodiazepines: actions

"**BenSCAM**s Pam into seduction **not by brain** but by muscle":
Sedation
anti-Convulsant
anti-Anxiety
Muscle relaxant
Not by brain: No antipsychotic activity.

Beta 1 selective blockers
"**BEAM ONE** up, Scotty":
Beta 1 blockers:
Esmolol
Atenolol
Metropolol

Botulism toxin: action, related bungarotoxin
Action: "**Bo**tulism **Bo**ttles up the Ach so it can't be the released":
Related bungarotoxin: "**B**otulism is related to **B**eta **B**ungarotoxin (beta-, not alpha-bungarotoxin--alpha has different mechanism).
Cholinergics (eg organophosphates): effects
If you know these, you will be "**LESS DUMB**":
Lacrimation
Excitation of nicotinic synapses
Salivation
Sweating
Diarrhea
Urination
Micturition
Bronchoconstriction

Delerium-causing drugs
ACUTE CHANGE IN MS:
Antibiotics (biaxin, penicillin, ciprofloxacin)
Cardiac drugs (digoxin, lidocaine)
Urinary incontinence drugs (anticholinergics)
Theophylline
Ethanol
Corticosteroids
H2 blockers
Antiparkinsonian drugs

Narcotics (esp. mepridine)
Geriatric psychiatric drugs
ENT drugs
Insomnia drugs
NSAIDs (eg indomethacin, naproxin)
Muscle relaxants
Seizure medicines

Direct sympathomimetic catecholamines

DINED:

Dopamine
Isoproterenol
Norepinephrine
Epinephrine
Dobutamine

Inhalation anesthetics

SHINE:

Sevoflurane
Halothane
Isoflurane
Nitrous oxide
Enflurane

If want the defunct **M**ethoxyflurane too, make it **MoonSHINE**.

Ipratropium: action

Atropine is buried in the middle: ipr**Atropi**um, so it behaves like Atropine.

Lead poisoning: presentation

ABCDEFG:

Anemia
Basophilic stripping

Colicky pain
Diarrhea
Encephalopathy
Foot drop
Gum (lead line)

Lithium: side effects
LITH:
Leukocytosis
Insipidus [diabetes insipidus, tied to polyuria]
Tremor/ Teratogenesis
Hypothyroidism

MAOIs: indications
MAOI'S:
Melancholic [classic name for atypical depression]
Anxiety
Obesity disorders [anorexia, bulemia]
Imagined illnesses [hypochondria]
Social phobias
   Listed in decreasing order of importance.
   Note MAOI is inside MelAnchOlIc.

Methyldopa: side effects
METHYLDOPA:
Mental retardation
Electrolyte imbalance
Tolerance
Headache/ Hepatotoxicity
psYcological upset
Lactation in female
Dry mouth
Oedema

Parkinsonism
Anaemia (haemolytic)

Monoamine oxidase inhibitors: members
"**PIT** of despair":
Phenelzine
Isocarboxazid
Tranylcypromine
　A pit of despair, since MAOs treat depression.

Morphine: effects
MORPHINES:
Miosis
Orthostatic hypotension
Respiratory depression
Pain supression
Histamine release/ Hormonal alterations
Increased ICT
Nausea
Euphoria
Sedation

Morphine: effects at mu receptor
PEAR:
Physical dependence
Euphoria
Analgesia
Respiratory depression

Narcotic antagonists
The Narcotic Antagonists are **NA**loxone and **NA**ltrexone.
　Important clinically to treat narcotic overdose.

Parkinsonism: drugs

SALAD:

Selegiline

Anticholinenergics (trihexyphenidyl, benzhexol, ophenadrine)

L-Dopa + peripheral decarboxylase inhibitor (carbidopa, benserazide)

Amantadine

Dopamine postsynaptic receptor agonists (bromocriptine, lisuride, pergolide)

Phenytoin: adverse effects

PHENYTOIN:

P-450 interactions

Hirsutism

Enlarged gums

Nystagmus

Yellow-browning of skin

Teratogenicity

Osteomalacia

Interference with B12 metabolism (hence anemia)

Neuropathies: vertigo, ataxia, headache

Physostigmine vs. neostigmine

LMNOP:

Lipid soluble

Miotic

Natural

Orally absorbed well

Physostigmine

   Neostigmine, on the contrary, is:

Water soluble

Used in myesthenia gravis

Synthetic

Poor oral absorption

Pupils in overdose: morphine vs. amphetamine

"Mor**PHINE**: **Fine**. Am**PHET**amine: **Fat**":

Mor**phine** overdose: pupils constricted (**fine**).

Am**phet**amine overdose: pupils dilated (**fat**).

Serotonin syndrome: components

Causes **HARM**:

Hyperthermia

Autonomic instability (delirium)

Rigidity

Myoclonus

Sodium valproate: side effects

VALPROATE:

Vomiting

Alopecia

Liver toxicity

Pancreatitis/ **P**ancytopenia

Retention of fats (weight gain)

Oedema (peripheral oedema)

Appetite increase

Tremor

Enzyme inducer (liver)

SSRIs: side effects

SSRI:

Serotonin syndrome

Stimulate CNS

Reproductive disfunctions in male

Insomnia

Succinylcholine: action, use

Succinylcholine gets **Stuck** to Ach receptor, then **Suck**s ions in through open pore.

You **Suck** stuff in through a mouth-tube, and drug is used for intubation.

Tricyclic antidepressants: members worth knowing

"I have to hide, the **CIA** is after me":

Clomipramine
Imipramine
Amitrptyline

If want the next 3 worth knowing, the **DND**is also after me:

Desipramine
Norrtriptyline
Doxepin

Tricyclic antidipressents (TCA): side effects

TCA'S:

Thrombocytopenia
Cardiac (arrhymia, MI, stroke)
Anticholinergic (tachycardia, urinary retention, etc)
Seizures

Vigabatrin: mechanism

Vi-GABA-Tr-In:

Via **GABAT**ransferase **In**hibition

Antibiotics contraindicated during pregnancy

MCAT:

Metronidazole
Chloramphenicol
Aminoglycoside
Tetracycline

Busulfan: features

ABCDEF:

Alkylating agent

Bone marrow suppression s/e

CML indication

Dark skin (hyperpigmentation) s/e

Endrocrine insufficiency (adrenal) s/e

Fibrosis (pulmonary) s/e

Cancer drugs: time of action between DNA->mRNA

ABCDEF:

Alkylating agents

Bleomycin

Cisplastin

Dactinomycin/ **D**oxorubicin

Etoposide

Flutamide and other steroids or their antagonists (eg tamoxifen, leuprolide)

Etoposide: action, indications, side effect

"e**TOP**oside":

  Action:

Inhibits **TOP**oisomerase II

  Indications:

Testicular carcinoma

Oat cell carcinoma of lung

Prostate carcinoma

  Side effect:

Affects **TOP** of your head, causing **alopecia**

Metabolism enzyme inducers

"Randy's Black Car Goes Putt Putt and Smokes":

Rifampin
Barbiturates
Carbamazepine
Grisoefulvin
Phenytoin
Phenobarb
Smoking cigarettes

Morphine: side-effects

MORPHINE:

Myosis
Out of it (sedation)
Respiratory depression
Pneumonia (aspiration)
Hypotension
Infrequency (constipation, urinary retention)
Nausea
Emesis

Therapeutic index: formula

TILE:

TI = LD50 / ED50

Torsades de Pointes: drugs causing

APACHE:

Amiodarone
Procainamide
Arsenium
Cisapride
Haloperidol
Eritromycin

Zero order kinetics drugs (most common ones)

"**PEAZ** (sounds like pees) out a constant amount":

Phenytoin

Ethanol

Aspirin

Zero order

  Someone that pees out a constant amount describes zero order kinetics (always the same amount out)

Asthma drugs: leukotriene inhibitor action

z**A**firlukast: **A**ntagonist of lipoxygenase

z**I**lueton: **I**nhibitor of LT receptor

Beta-1 vs Beta-2 receptor location

"You have **1 heart** and **2 lungs**":

Beta-**1** are therefore primarily on **heart**.

Beta-**2** primarily on **lungs**.

Respiratory depression inducing drugs

"**STOP** breathing":

Sedatives and hypnotics

Trimethoprim

Opiates

Polymyxins

Ribavirin: indications

RIBAvirin:

RSV

Influenza **B**

Arenaviruses (Lassa, Bolivian, etc.)

TB: antibiotics used
STRIPE:

STreptomycin

Rifampicin

Isoniazid

Pyrizinamide

Ethambutol

Zafirlukast, Montelukast, Cinalukast: mechanism, usage
"Zafir-**luk-ast**, Monte-**luk-ast**, Cina-**luk-ast**":

Anti-**Luk**otrienes for **Ast**hma.

Dazzle your oral examiner: Za**fir**lukast antagonizes leukotriene-**4**.

Teratogenic drugs: major non-antibiotics
TAP CAP:

Thalidomide

Androgens

Progestins

Corticosteroids

Aspirin & indomethacin

Phenytoin

Tetracycline: teratogenicity
TEtracycline is a

TEratogen that causes staining of

TEeth in the newborn.

Antirheumatic agents (disease modifying): members
CHAMP:

Cyclophosphamide

Hydroxycloroquine and choloroquinine

Auranofin and other gold compounds

Methotrexate

Penicillamine

Auranofin, aurothioglucose: category and indication

Aurum is latin for "gold" (gold's chemical symbol is **Au**).
Generic Aur- drugs (**Aur**anofin, **Aur**othioglucose) are gold
compounds.

If didn't learn yet that gold's indication is rheumatoid arthritis,
AUR- **A**cts **U**pon**R**heumatoid.

PHYSICS

Ideal gas law

"**P**ure **V**irgins **N**ever **R**eally **T**ire":
$PV = nRT$

Ohm's Law

"**V**irgins **A**re **R**are":
Volts = **A**mps x **R**esistance

Note: can then rearrange to more common form Resistance = Volts
/ Amps.

Work: formula

"Lots of **Work** gets me **Mad**!":
Work = Mad:
M=**M**ass
a=**a**cceleration
d=**d**istance

Carotid sinus vs. carotid body function

carotidSinuS: measures preSSure.

carotid bO2dy measures **O2**.

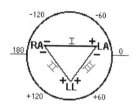

Einthoven's Triangle: organization

Corners are at RA (right arm), LA (left arm), **LL** (left leg).

Number of L's at a corner tell how many + signs are at that corner [eg **LL** is ++].

Sum of number of L's of any 2 corners tells the name of the lead [eg **LL-LA** is lead**III**].

For reference axes, the **negative angle** hemisphere is on the half of the triangle drawing that has all the

negative signs; **positive angle** hemisphere contains only **positive signs**.

Hb-oxygen dissociation curve shifts: effect, location

Left shift: causes Loading of O2 in Lungs.

Right shift: causes Release of O2 from Hb.

Heart electrical conduction pathway

"If patient's family are all having **Heart** attacks, you must **SAVe HIS KIN!**"

SA node --->

AV node --->

His (bundle of) -->

Pur**KIN**je fibers

Intrinsic vs. extrinsic pathway tests

"Pe**T**Pi**TT**bull":

Pe**T**: **PT** is for extrinsic pathway.

Pi**TT**bull: **PTT** is for intrinsic pathway.

PGI2 vs. TxA2 coagulation function

TxA2 Aggregates platelets.

PGI2 Inhibits aggregation.

Note: full name of PGI2 is prostaglandin I2 or prostacyclin, full name of TxA2 is thromboxane A2.

Adrenal cortex layers and products

"Go Find Rex, Make Good Sex":

Layers:

Glomerulosa

Fasiculata

Reticulata

Respective products:

Mineralcorticoids

Glucocorticoids

Sex hormones

Alternatively for layers: GFR (Glomerular Filtration Rate, convenient since adrenal glands are atop kidney).

Adrenal gland: functions

ACTH:

Adrenergic functions

Catabolism of proteins/ Carbohydrate metabolism

T cell immunomodulation

Hyper/ Hypotension (blood pressure control)

Diabetes Insipidous: diagnosing subtypes

After a desmopression injection:

Concentrated urine = Cranial.

No effect = Nephrogenic.

Hyperthyroidism: signs and symptoms

THYROIDISM:

Tremor
Heart rate up
Yawning [fatigability]
Restlessness
Oligomenorrhea & amenorrhea
Intolerance to heat
Diarrhea
Irritability
Sweating
Musle wasting & weight loss

Pituitary hormones
FLAGTOP:
Follicle stimulating hormone
Lutinizing hormone
Adrenocorticotropin hormone
Growth hormone
Thyroid stimulating hormone
Oxytocin
Prolactin
Alternatively: **GOAT FLAP** with the second 'A' for **A**nti-diruetic homone/vasopressin
Note: there is also melanocyte secreting homone and Lipotropin, but they are not well understood.

Progesterone: actions
PROGESTE:
Produce cervical mucous
Relax uterine smooth muscle
Oxycotin sensitivity down
Gonadotropin [FSH, LH] secretions down
Endometrial spiral arteries and secretions up
Sustain pregnancy

Temperature up / Tit development
Excitability of myometrium down

Balance organs
Utricle and Saccule keep **US** balanced.

Temperature control: cerebral regions
"**H**igh **P**ower **A**ir **C**onditioner":
Heating = **P**osterior hipothalamo [hypothalamus].
Anterior hipothalamo [hypothalamus] = **C**ooling.

Urination: autonomic control
"When you pee, it's **PIS**s":
Parasympathetic **I**nhibits **S**ympathetic.

Alkalosis vs. acidosis: directions of pH and HCO3
ROME:
Respiratory= **O**pposite:
   pH is high, PCO2 is down (Alkalosis).
   pH is low, PCO2 is up (Acidosis).
Metabolic= **E**qual:
   pH is high, HCO3 is high (Alkalosis).
   pH is low, HCO3 is low (Acidosis).

Compliance of lungs factors
COMPLIANCE:
Collagen deposition (fibrosis)
Ossification of costal cartilages
Major obesity
Pulmonary venous congestion
Lung size
Increased expanding pressure
Age

No surfactant
Chest wall scarring
Emphysema
   All but L/A/E decrease compliance.

V/Q gradient in lung
   Infinity, a lung and a zero stack nicely.
   V/Q is lowest at bottom, highest at top.
   See diagram.

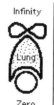

Infinity

Zero

Also, a **shunt** is "**O**" shaped at end so V/Q=**O** is a **shunt**.
And when you are **dead** you go into the **great beyond**, so anatomical **dead** space is V/Q=**infinity**.

Prolactin and oxytocin: functions
   PROlactin stimulates the mammary glands to **PRO**duce milk.
   Oxytocin stimulates the mammary glands to **O**oze (release) milk.

Osteoblast vs. osteoclast
   Osteo**B**last **B**uilds bone.
   Osteo**C**last **C**onsumes bone.

PODIATRY

Blue toe (microembolic toe)
   CAVEMAN:
   Cholesterol embolizations
   Atrial fib with electricity or digitoxin
   Valvular problems
   Endocarditis
   Mural thrimbosis
   Aneurysm/ **A**V fistula
   Nothing

TIA: internal carotid vs. vertebrobasilar
   MD vs. DPM
      Internal carotid:

Monocular blindness (amaurox fugax)
Dominant hemisphere (apahsia)
  The weakness or numbness is still less in the legs.
  Vetebrobasilar:
Diplopia/ Double blindness
Paralysis (quadriplesia)
Motor weakness (ipsilateral)
  Ataxia is characteristic in veterbrobasilar lesions.

Diabetic neuropathy types
  DPM:
  Distal, symmetric, polyneuropathy
  Proximal diabetic neuropathy
  Mononeuritis muliplex

Arthritides: the six classifications
  "Round **COINS**":
  Rheumatoid diseases (inflammation of synovium)
  Crystal depositions (gout, pseudogout)
  Osteoarthritis
  Infections
  Neuropathy
  SLE, mixed scleroderma

Charcot's joints: common disorders
  "Come See **AHan**dsome **DPM**":
  Congenital insenisitivity to pain
  Syringomyelia/ Spina bifida
  Alcoholism
  Hansen's disease
  Diabetes mellitus
  Peripheral nerve injury
  Menigomyelocele

Dialysis: indications

AEIOU:
Acid-base problems (severe acidosis or alkalosis)
Electrolyte problems (hyperkalemia)
Intoxications
Overload, fluid
Uremic symptoms

Enlarged kidneys: causes

SHAPE:
Sclerderma
HIV nephropathy
Amyloidosis
Polycystic kidney disease
Endocrinophathy (diabetes)

Hematuria: differential

SHIT:
Stones/ Systemic disease (SLE)/ Structural lesions (UPJ obstruction)
Hematologic disease (sickle cell, coagulopathy)/ Hypercalciuria/
Hereditary (Alport nephritis)/ HSP/ HUS
Infectious and Immunologic (PSGN)/ IgA nephropathy (Berger
nephritis)/ Interstitial disease (interstitial nephritis)/ Idiopathic
conditions(thin glomerular basement membrane disease or benign
familial hematuria)
Trauma/ Tumor/ TB/ Toxins

Hydronephrosis: differential

Unilateral is **PACT**:
Pelvic-uteric obstruction (congenital or acquired)
Aberrant renal vessels
Calculi
Tumours of renal pelvis
Bilateral is **SUPER**:
Stenosis of the urethra
Urethral valve
Prostatic enlargement
Extensive bladder tumour
Retro-peritoneal fibrosis

Nephrotic syndrome: causes for secondary nephrotic syndrome

DAVID:
Diabetes mellitus
Amyloidosis
Vasculitis
Infections
Drugs

Polycystic kidney: genetic marker

"**P**" is the **16**th letter of the alphabet.
Autosomal dominant **P**olycystic kidney disease is associated with abberation on the **16**th chromosome.

Prostatism: initial symptoms

"Prostatism is initially **FUN**":
Frequency
Urgency
Nocturia

Pyelonephritis (acute): predisposing factors

SCARRIN' UP:
Sex (females <40, males >40)
Catheterization
Age (infant, elderly)
Renal lesions
Reflux (vesciouteral)
Immunodeficienct
NIDDM, IDDM
Urinary obstuction
Pregnant
Acute pyelonephritis heals by scarrin' up the area (pyelonephritic scar).

Urinary incontinence: causes of acute and reversible

DRIP:
Delirium
Restricted mobility/ **R**etention
Inflammation / **I**nfection/ **I**mpaction [fecal]
Pharmaceuticals / **P**olyuria
"Drip" is convenient since it is urinary incontinence, so urine only drips out.

Testicular atrophy: differential

TESTES SHRINK:

Trauma
Exhaustional atrophy
Sequelae
Too little food
Elderly
Semen obstruction
Sex hormone therapy
Hypopituitarism
Radiation
Inflammatory orchitis
Not descended
Kleinfelter's

SURGERY

Fistulas: conditions preventing closure

FRIEND:

Foreign body
Radiation
Infection/ Inflammation (Crohn)
Epithelialization
Neoplasia
Distal obstruction

Oesophageal cancer risk factors

PC BASTARDS:

Plummer-Vinson syndrome
Coeliac disease
Barrett's
Alcohol
Smoking
Tylosis
Achalasia
Russia (geographical distribution)
Diet

GI bleeding: causes

ABCDEFGHI:
Angiodysplasia
Bowel cancer
Colitis
Diverticulitis/ Duodenal ulcer
Epitaxis/ Esophageal (cancer, esophagitis, varices)
Fistula (anal, aortaenteric)
Gastric (cancer, ulcer, gastritis)
Hemorrhoids
Infectious diarrhoea/ IBD/ Ischemic bowel

Varicose veins: symptoms

AEIOU:
Aching
Eczema
Itching
Oedema
Ulceration/ Ugly (LDS, haemosiderin, varicosities)

Melanoma sites

"**Mel SEA**" (Pronounced "Mel C" from the Spice Girls)
   Melanoma sites, in order of frequency:
Skin
Eyes
Anus

Post-operative fever causes

Six W's:
Wind: pulmonary system is primary source of fever first 48 hours, may have pneumonia
Wound: infection at surgical site
Water: check IV for phlebitis
Walk: deep venous thrombosis, due to pelvic pooling or restricted mobility related to pain and fatigue
Whiz: urinary tract infection if urinary catheterization
Wonder drugs: drug-induced fever

Appendicectomy: complications

WRAP IF HOT:
Wound infection
Respiratory (atelectasis, pneumonia)
Abscess (pelvic)
Portal pyemia
Ileus (paralytic)
Fecal fistula
Hernia (r. inguinal)
Obstruction (intestinal due to adhesions)
Thrombus (DVT)

Post-operative complications (immediate)

"Post-op **PROBS**":
Pain
Primary haemorrhage
Reactionary haemorrhage
Oliguria
Basal atelectasis
Shock/ Sepsis

Compartment syndrome: signs and symptoms

5 P's:
Pain
Palor
P ulseless
Paresethesia
Pressure (increased)

RHEUMATOLOGY /ALLERGY

SLE (Systemic Lupus Erythematosus) diagnosis

"**MD SOAP 'N HAIR**":
Malar rash
Discoid rash
Serositis
Oral ulcer
Arthritis
Photosensitivity
Neurologic abnormality
Hematologic abnormality

ANA (+)
Immunologic abnormality
Renal involvement

Felty's syndrome: components

SANTA:
Splenomegaly
Anaemia
Neutropenia
Thrombocytopenia
Arthritis (rheumatoid)

Carpal tunnel syndrome

TINel's sign:
TINgling sensation after
Tapping on
Traumatized nerve in carpal
Tunnel syndrome

Henoch schonlein purpura: signs and symptoms

NAPA:
Nephritis
Arthritis, arthralgias
Purpura, palpable (especially on buttocks and lower extremities)
Abdominal pain (need to rule out intussusception)

Asthma: treatment

ASTHMA:
Adrenergics
Steroids
Theophylline
Hydration
Mask [O2 at 24%]
Antibiotics

Arthritis: juvenile idiopathic: differential

ARTHRITIS:
Anxiety
Rickets and metabolic
Tumor
Hematological
Reactive arthritis
Immunological (SLE)
Trauma

Injury
Sepsis

Arthritis: seronegative spondyloarthropathies

PEAR:
Psoriatic arthritis
Enteropathic arthritis
Ankylosing sponylitis
Reiter's/ Reactive

Joint pain causes

SOFTER TISSUE:
Sepsis
Osteoarthritis
Fractures
Tendon/muscle
Epiphyseal
Referred
Tumor
Ischaemia
Seropositive arthritides
Seronegative arthritides
Urate
Extra-articular rheumatism (such as polymylagia)

Osteoporosis risk factors

ACCESS:
Alcohol
Corticosteroid
Calcium low
Estrogen low
Smoking
Sedentary lifestyle

Made in the USA
Middletown, DE
07 June 2016